HOW TO
THRIVE
PAST 55

HOW TO THRIVE PAST 55

EDITED BY
DEANNA WILSON

HELP THE AGED

LIFEGUIDES

EDITOR

Deanna Wilson, who revised and expanded the text of this book for the LifeGuides series, is an award-winning journalist and editor based in London, specialising in healthcare, medicine and related topics. She edits *Women's Health Today*, which is published on behalf of the National Association of Primary Care and distributed through GP surgeries.

LifeGuides are commissioned and published by Help the Aged, 207–221 Pentonville Road, London N1 9UZ and can be purchased via www.helptheaged.org.uk or from bookshops

For a full list of Help the Aged publications, see the website, telephone 020 7239 1946 or email publications@helptheaged.org.uk.

First published 2008

Copyright © 2008 Help the Aged

Trade distribution by Turnaround Publisher Services Ltd

British Library Cataloguing in Publication Data
A catalogue record for this book is available from the British Library

ISBN 978-1-84598-029-0

Designed and typeset by Price Watkins Design
Printed and bound in England by CPI Mackay Ltd

CONTENTS

CONTENTS, continued

1

THE AMAZING TRUTH ABOUT AGEING

THE AMAZING TRUTH ABOUT AGEING

I f you are a 55-year-old reading this book, you may be interested to know that you can expect to live, on average, another 24 years (for men) or 26 years (for women). But most of us have probably got our sights set higher than mere survival. We want to have the health and vitality to enjoy our later years. So what can we do to make sure that our fitness lasts as long as we do — in other words, to enjoy not just a full life span, but a full health span?

If you are old enough to be reading this book, you are old enough to know how you want to live your life. But the fact that you are reading it at all suggests that you are interested in your own health as you get older, and possibly in that of members of your family too. We have all seen that older age can be bleak for some: disabilities and difficulties can eat away at people's quality of life. Equally, we have all come across the sprightly 80- or 90-year-olds who do their own shopping, gardening and entertaining and are active in the local community. Can we do anything to improve our chances of coming in the second group and avoiding the first?

The answer is a resounding 'yes'. This book is packed with good news about simple things we can do to maximise our chances of a healthy and active older age. What is more, science shows that **it is never too late to make a change in lifestyle that will benefit our health.** So whether you are 55 or 85, you can start making a difference today.

HEALTH ADVICE: WHAT SHOULD WE BELIEVE?

Nowadays it is hard to avoid health advice. It screams at us from newspapers, magazines, radio and TV, health-food shops, the internet, even the supermarket. Some of this advice is sound and sensible, but some is not. How do we know which we can trust and which we should take with a large pinch of salt? Much of it claims to be based on 'research' ('studies of Megaherb have shown it can knock years off your age'). 'Research', however, means different things to different people and much of it is deeply flawed, or carried out in order to provide some sort of justification for a marketing claim. It is also worrying that, for example, anyone can call themselves a 'nutritionist' and promote the likes of Megaherb without anything to back up their assertions.

This book is about what science tells us about how to age successfully. Every statement we make here is backed up by the most rigorous research currently available. If some finding is not yet proven, or is controversial, we say so. Science has a unique contribution to make to our understanding of ageing. It can shed light on the links with lifestyle and genes, as well as pioneering treatments that can help us in later life. Our aim is to give you the most reliable, scientific information about ageing so you can make informed decisions about your lifestyle.

That said, we have to add an important note about the nature of the evidence in medical science. Much science is based on the observation of large populations and their health patterns. For example, studies have revealed that vegetarians have lower rates of cancer and heart disease than meat-eaters. But is this because they do not eat meat or because they eat more vegetables than the average meat-eater? Are other factors at work? The risks for cancer, as for any other disease, are complex and are unlikely to be explained by one factor alone. Do vegetarians run health risks that these particular studies did not ask about? Observational findings have to be regarded as generating ideas rather than proving them.

Some of the advice in this book has to be based on observational studies because the further research that we need remains to be done. Research into Ageing, the biomedical research programme at Help the Aged, is working hard to fund research, but we also want others to appreciate the significance of this missing information.

The science of ageing is still in its infancy and most experts agree that there is a lot we do not know – which is why Research into Ageing has such a heavy workload. However, we believe that what you will read here is robust enough to stand the test of time. Nutritionists have been saying for at least 30 years that we should eat more fruit and vegetables and what the newest studies are showing are yet more reasons why this is valuable advice.

So you will probably already know some of the things you read in this book. But we are confident that some of the findings will surprise – and even delight – you.

WHAT IS AGEING?

People who are researching the phenomenon of ageing are taking a close look at our cells, and particularly at the mechanisms that may damage them. Experts believe that way back in history, when life was precarious and people could expect to live only to about 30 – because at any time they could be overwhelmed by infection, illness, accident or starvation – evolution was essentially geared to ensuring that we passed on our genes to the next generation. As a result, our sex cells have high-quality protection mechanisms, but the other cells in our body, the somatic (body) cells are more disposable in the great evolutionary scheme, and are given lower priority by the body's systems for maintenance and repair, which include DNA repair, antioxidant defences and protein turnover.

According to Professor Tom Kirkwood, it was really a kind of trade-off to ensure the survival of the human race. But because people died so young, it meant that cell mutations in early life that produced adverse effects at later ages were not eliminated from the gene pool. The upshot for us is that ageing is the result of a lifelong accumulation of faults at the cellular and molecular levels. 'Each of these faults may individually be unimportant,' he explains, 'but eventually they build up in such numbers that they overwhelm the body's capacity to keep its life support systems running.'

The good news about this theory is that by studying how to support the repair and maintenance functions of the cell, we can do much to improve how we age and to ensure that we live as long as possible, free of the disabling conditions that can undermine the quality of our later life.

For instance, a great deal of research concerns antioxidants and whether they can prevent cell damage, disease and ageing. They work by mopping up the toxins called free radicals which are produced continuously in our body through the natural process of oxidation, which turns oxygen into energy. With time, though, the process becomes less efficient, and free radical damage has been implicated in several age-related conditions, such as Alzheimer's, cancer and heart disease.

The other main threat to our health in later life comes from invasion by bacteria or viruses, or by cancer cells, when cells grow out of control. In fact, we are regularly assailed by these threats throughout life, but as long as our immune system is in good order its armies of differently specialised defence cells successfully destroy the invaders. Unfortunately, our immune system declines with age and becomes less effective. As a result, we become more prone to infections, and take longer to recover.

As yet, the scientists are agreed that eating fruit, vegetables and other plant compounds such as green tea, ginger, garlic, turmeric and chilli, which all contain antioxidants, can help reduce our risk of these diseases. But the jury is still out on whether taking antioxidant supplements is helpful. A recent study found that the promising results found in the lab were simply not reproduced in the human body. None the less, some experts believe that supplements can be helpful, particularly for older people, who may be unable for whatever reason to obtain optimal levels of nutrients from their food. So we are still a long way from a definitive answer. Meanwhile, make sure you aim for your five portions of fruit and vegetables a day.

And that's what this book is all about – a guide to measures you can take to keep yourself in good health, or to manage a long-term condition, based on scientifically validated evidence.

MAKING THE RIGHT CHOICES

Today, we have much safer and longer lives than our ancestors did. The health risks we face have moved on. We do have to be wary of some external elements over which we have little direct control as individuals – the effect of environmental pollutants on our health is one example. But the main spotlight now is on our lifestyle, as the key driver in what happens to our health, more influential even than the genes we were born with.

And that gives us choices. There is a huge amount of interest in health matters – healthcare sites are the second most popular on the internet. Yet the underlying message for good health is very straightforward. What we have to do is be aware of our lifestyle and be willing to make adjustments to it if necessary. What we eat and drink matters. Exercise matters. Staying in touch with people matters. So does having a laugh every day.

Actress Joan Collins has plenty of tips for the rest of us. At 74, she gave *The Mail on Sunday* her recipe for growing old gracefully. 'I tell all the women I meet, look after your skin and eat less. You need half the amount of food at 50 as you ate at 25. But don't diet – it's really bad for your skin. If your skin looks on the way out, eat a ton of olive oil, like I do. Never drink tap water. I have an aversion to drinking recycled urine and hormones. Exercise a little and you'll always look much younger than your age. Do think about HRT, when the time comes. Did it work for me? Er, helloooo… Oh, and never fall and break your hip. There's nothing more ageing than a Zimmer frame.' ∎

2

MAKING THE MOST OF OUR LONGER LIVES

MAKING THE MOST OF
OUR LONGER LIVES

We are definitely living longer and enjoying good health for longer than ever before. Who says so? Well, the government's actuaries for one – and they are not a breed given to exaggeration – since the official retirement age is to be extended to 66 in 2030, 67 in 2040 and 68 in 2050, with the option of going as high as 69. For women, the state pension age will rise from 60 to 65 by 2020.

Meanwhile, life expectancy is increasing exponentially. In 1980, for example, a 65-year-old woman typically lived for a further 18 years, but the government expects this to rise to 22 years by 2020 and to 26 years by 2050. Although men continue to lag behind, the gap is definitely narrowing. Figures from the Office for National Statistics in 2007 suggest that the average woman can expect to live to 81, the average man to 79. And, say the actuaries, a man aged 50 in 2007 who reaches 65 can thereafter expect to live until nearly 90.

Of course, some of this is thanks to improved medical treatments which are enabling people to survive major disease. Some types of heart disease and cancer, for example, are increasingly seen as chronic diseases, and not the acute killers they once were. Indeed, deaths occurring at under age 75 are nowadays considered premature.

So the big question becomes 'How do we add life to years, to get the most out of every day?'.

THE KEYS TO A LONGER LIFESPAN

A recent online consumer survey run by the insurer Legal & General showed that we do have a handle on how to go about it. Respondents thought that improving lifestyle would do far more to improve lifespan than relying on medical intervention. The best routes are seen as:

- taking regular exercise (72 per cent)
- having a healthier diet (63 per cent) and
- leading a less stressful life (49 per cent)

– precisely what the doctor would order.

But it does not yet mean that we are all actually practising what we preach. How else can we explain that the rate of obesity in the United Kingdom has more than tripled over the past 20 years, according to OECD figures for 2006?

Thankfully, though, it has got much easier to judge for oneself whether one is obese or not.

The BMI (body mass index), a system of measurement first developed in 1832, is on its way out, basically because it does not differentiate between lean muscle mass and fat and therefore cannot indicate risks or progress in an individual.

Nowadays, the emphasis is turning to where precisely the extra fat is stored, and this is bringing in new ways of measuring obesity. Fat accumulates under the skin and around the vital organs in the abdomen. People who are apple-shaped have more fat around the tummy than on their hips and bottom. If the reverse is true, then they are pear-shaped. A large amount of fat around the abdomen increases the risk of heart problems, diabetes, high blood pressure and stroke, and can play havoc with metabolism. So the advice nowadays is to measure obesity via your waist.

For women, the ideal waist size is less than 80cm (32 in); high is 80–88cm (32–35 in), and very high over 88cm (35 in). For men, the ideal is less than 94 cm (37 in); high is 94–102cm (37–40 in), and very high is more than 88cm (35 in). To find your waist-to-hip ratio, measure your hips, then your waist, and divide the waist number by the hip number. For a healthy woman, the total should be under 0.85. For a man it should be below 0.90.

Now, a much more sophisticated system that can measure precisely where mass and body fat are stored in the body, and relate this to factors such as height and medical risk, is being tried out in the NHS. The Body Benchmark Study is based on using a 3-D scanner to measure a person in less than seven seconds. It does not involve radiation and it is not invasive. The hope is that it will eventually evolve into an internationally recognised Body Volume Index (BVI) to replace the BMI, giving far more accurate results and providing a motivational tool in treating obesity and eating disorders.

A JOURNEY OF DISCOVERY

Never before in history have so many people lived so long, which means there is still a lot to find out about their health and lifestyles. Increasingly, the tools that are being used for this are large-scale surveys that are repeated over time with the same people. One such is the ELSA study (the English Longitudinal Study of Ageing), which charts the situation of some 9,000 people every two years. The overall idea is to help guide government policies on services for older people.

The latest ELSA report, for 2005, presents a somewhat mixed bag. On the one hand, more than half of those aged 65 or older considered their health good or very good. On the other, 65 per cent of women and 48 per cent of men found it difficult to walk up a flight of 12 stairs without resting. Some 23 per cent of men and 29 per cent of women had fallen in the previous 12 months. Cardiovascular disease was the most common chronic disease among men (37 per cent), while arthritis was the most common chronic disease in women (47 per cent). Almost two-thirds of the group had high blood pressure (hypertension), and 22 per cent had visited their GP in the previous two weeks. Finally, when rated on a scale measuring general levels of happiness, depression and anxiety, sleep disturbance and the ability to cope, 12 per cent of women and 9 per cent of men reported low levels of psychosocial well-being.

The chapters that follow will be taking a more detailed look at what can be done to prevent or manage these health problems.

There is also a new form of self-help for people living with long-term conditions, in the shape of local self-management courses. The scheme is being run on behalf of local primary care trusts (PCTs) by the newly established Expert Patient Programme Community Interest Company (EPP CIC), and includes training volunteers to run local courses. The thinking is that if people know how best to manage a chronic condition, this will reduce the likelihood of their needing emergency care. Already, A&E attendances are down by more than 15 per cent among people who have attended a course. Now, the aim is to increase the number of course places every year, from 12,000 in 2007 to 100,000 by 2012.

Further practical help is available to people who are of pensionable age, disabled or suffering from long-term health problems, by calling the Home Heat Helpline (see chapter 10) for access to a range of benefits and advice. For instance, special controls and adaptors can be supplied to older people having trouble using certain appliances, meters that are in an inconvenient position can be moved, and people can get help with their energy bills. The service is funded by Britain's six main energy suppliers.

ALL IN THE GENES ...

For most of us, 60 really is the new 40. It helps, of course, if you chose your parents carefully and were born with a good stock of genes. Also, according to Professor Tim Skerry of the University of Sheffield, it helps if you moved about a lot in the womb. These brief periods of activity seem to promote normal bone mass and our skeletal architecture, suggesting that whether or not we develop bone disease in later life is at least partly determined while we are still a foetus.

As far as the contribution of our genes to our health is concerned, we now know that a genetic tendency underlies just about every disorder. But we need to get away from the idea that a single gene (or the lack of it) is likely to be responsible for a specific disease. This applies to only a very few conditions, cystic fibrosis and sickle-cell anaemia among them.

Much more often, it is a matter of inheriting a clutch of related genes that work together to produce disease when triggered by outside factors such as infection, chronic inflammation, or environmental pollutants. A great deal of current basic scientific research is focused on identifying these clusters of genes and the sorts of triggers that set them off.

Interestingly, Parkinson's disease is a condition where both types of gene mechanisms can be found. Whereas a single gene is involved in the 10 per cent of sufferers who have the hereditary form, a cluster of related genes has now been discovered that could account for some 70 per cent of cases. There is also some evidence that the cause may lie in a combination of genes and a farm upbringing.

Parkinson's disease (PD) occurs when a small part of the brain known as the substantia nigra (black nucleus), which has an important role in enabling the smooth flow of movement, is damaged. As a result, less of the neurotransmitter dopamine is produced. Symptoms, which often appear gradually but become increasingly severe, include tremors; difficulty in maintaining balance and gait; rigidity or stiffness, and general slowness of movement.

In the UK there are estimated to be 120,000 people with Parkinson's disease, and the condition is becoming much more common in people over 65. As yet, there is no cure, but stem-cell research and gene therapy are the treatment prospects being followed.

Given the way that medicines research is going, we can expect further progress in recognising different classes of genotypes. These are caused by polymorphisms – subtle variations to a particular gene that can be found in our DNA. The effect is to create subgroups of people who will benefit from a medication, and others for whom it might be actually harmful. One example comes from giving omega-3 immediately after a first heart attack. This has been found to reduce the risk of a second attack – depending on your genotype.

TECHNOLOGICAL ADVANCES

Other developments are dramatically altering the services available to us. If we do fall ill, for example, we can expect diagnosis and treatment to be far less invasive than ever before. Diagnosis has been greatly aided by the huge advances in imaging techniques that have been coming in over the last few years, leading to much-improved cure rates if the condition is picked up early enough.

Many types of operation have been transformed by the increasing use of minimally-invasive surgery, which involves very small incisions, or is carried out through a body cavity or anatomical opening. It can reduce the risk of post-operative complications and often enables the patient to leave hospital much sooner than in the past.

One area that has so far tended to lag behind is cancer surgery, with only about 5 per cent of patients treated through this approach, but we can expect to see it catching up with the overall trend.

Keyhole surgery is also making its mark in some types of hip and knee replacements, accompanied by a drive to improve the function and longevity of the implants themselves. One result is that implants for women are now being shaped to a woman's smaller size and to reflect the fact that women swivel their hips when walking, which men do not.

It is also worth bearing in mind that certain conditions (or stages thereof) benefit from doctors taking a 'watch and see' stance, so do not be put off if this happens to you. It is relatively common, for instance, for a woman found to have changes suggesting early cervical cancer to be checked again a few weeks later, and to find that the body has spontaneously sorted out the maverick cells. (She will go on being monitored for some time afterwards, just to be sure.)

SCREENING AND OTHER HEALTH CHECKS

Screening for various conditions is now upfront as never before, and we can expect a number of programmes to be added to the existing list. The NHS view is that screening should take place only where the evidence justifies it, as part of a national programme with standards, quality assurance and monitoring arrangements in place. Proposals for new screening programmes are considered by the UK National Screening Committee against a set of internationally recognised criteria to ensure that programmes do more good than harm at a reasonable cost.

Breast cancer screening is available through the NHS to all women aged between 50 and 70, and is carried out once every three years. Plans are in place to extend this to women aged 47–73. Women over 70 are not currently invited for screening, but can still have free mammograms every three years by making their own appointment.

Three-yearly cervical cancer screening – the smear test – starts at age 25, but from 50 to 65 the frequency switches to five-yearly. Women of 65 who have had three clear tests in a row are not recalled for further screening, as the risk is considered so low. But a woman of 65 or more who has never had a test is strongly urged to have one, even if she is no longer sexually active. The hope for the future is that the proposed introduction of a vaccine against cervical cancer, to be given to girls aged 12, will all but eradicate the disease and, eventually, do away with the need for a national screening programme.

As yet, there is no national screening programme for ovarian cancer, although trials currently under way are due to be completed in 2011. UKCTOCS, the United Kingdom Collaborative Trial of Ovarian Cancer Screening, is the largest such trial in the world, involving 200,000 randomly selected women at 12 centres around the UK.

The trial is testing two types of screening procedures which at present are only available in the private sector: a blood test looking for high levels of a protein called CA125, and vaginal ultrasound.

Meanwhile, a survey carried out by Ovarian Cancer Action has revealed a great deal of confusion between ovarian and cervical cancer in many people's minds. Some 45 per cent of women mistakenly believe that a smear test will indicate whether or not they have ovarian cancer, and 34 per cent mistakenly believe that the more sexual partners a woman has, the more this puts her at risk of ovarian cancer.

Two-thirds of women are unable to describe any symptoms of ovarian cancer, or say they do not know what the symptoms are, while 59 per cent say they do not know or are unable to mention any risk factors associated with ovarian cancer.

In fact, if you have recently started to experience one or more of the following symptoms, and they occur more than 12 times a month, make sure ovarian cancer is considered: feeling full, difficulty in eating, abdominal or pelvic pain, bloating, or increased abdominal size. It is the frequency and persistence that count.

Breast and cervical cancer screening have been available for some years, but the list now includes bowel cancer, chlamydia, and diabetic retinopathy (though not all are yet running on a fully national scale). There is also a push towards screening for vascular disease, which will include screening high-risk groups for Type 2 diabetes. It is likely that before too long we will have screening for abdominal aortic aneurysm, too, and, as already mentioned, ovarian cancer. Scanning plays a role in some of the approaches, but many utilise relatively low-key lab tests.

Interestingly, an element of self-referral is coming in with the chlamydia testing, aimed at preventing pelvic inflammatory disease. This is available in genito-urinary clinics or, for a small fee, in selected pharmacies, and is designed to encourage asymptomatic women and their partners to come forward. If you are back on the dating scene following a mid-life divorce, it is well worth checking yourself out. But the advice is to see your doctor rather than the pharmacist once you have hit 60.

Of course, if you work for a major organisation, you could well be the beneficiary of a company scheme offering MoT-style health checks via the private sector. The types of screening available, only privately to date, include carotid stenosis, testicular and ovarian cancer, and osteoporosis.

What other free NHS services are available to older people? Anyone aged 60 or over is entitled to free prescriptions and free NHS eye tests. Here, the recommended frequency is once every two years until you are 70, then once a year.

THE IMMUNE SYSTEM

Our bodies need protection from harmful invaders including bacteria, parasites and viruses, and sometimes also from their own cells, which may develop incorrectly (as happens with cancer cells). The immune system provides this protection through a series of barriers and toxic chemicals as well as a sophisticated system that can recognise, target and destroy unwelcome cells.

For example, your skin protects you against possible invaders by producing slightly acidic oil that controls the growth of things such as bacteria and fungi. The skin is also a physical barrier. If this is broken, it releases chemicals to signal that it needs help. This triggers an 'inflammatory response', which is a series of events involving:

- swelling to isolate the incoming bacteria
- white blood cells to destroy incoming bacteria
- enzymes to clear away the damaged tissue
- extra blood to help with healing, and
- specialist cells to rebuild and repair.

However, the inflammatory response may not be able to deal with all of the invaders. Some will probably slip through into the blood stream, where they will be dealt with by antibodies, which are produced by white blood cells. The antibodies are tailor-made to neutralise and destroy the bacteria.

A COMPLEX AND ADAPTABLE SYSTEM
The immune system is extremely complex: it can produce about 10

million different types of antibody to deal with the many possible invaders we can come into contact with. And because infection can spread very quickly, speed is always of the essence for the immune system.

To save time, the immune system files away a memory of every specific antibody that it makes. This means that the next time it encounters the same invader it will be able to quickly copy the correct antibody and thus destroy the invader as fast as possible. This defensive memory bank, known as acquired immunity, is the mechanism that enables us to use vaccination to protect ourselves from disease.

EVERYBODY MAKES MISTAKES
Sometimes the immune system makes a mistake and attacks its own body in the same way that it would normally attack a bacterium or virus. The result can be, for example:

- juvenile-onset diabetes, caused by the immune system eliminating the cells in the pancreas that produce insulin
- rheumatoid arthritis, caused by the immune system attacking tissues inside the joints.

Allergies are another example of the immune system getting it wrong. If you have an allergy to, say, pollen, your immune system is reacting to something that really should be ignored. It tries to wash out the 'invader' by making your nose run and eyes water. It also releases histamines to cause inflammation to help bring chemical defenders to the scene. You can override this false alarm by taking antihistamines.

THE IMMUNE SYSTEM IN LATER LIFE
Older cells tend to do most things more slowly. However, the immune system relies on rapid communication between cells as well as the speedy duplication of antibodies. Many of the components of the

immune system are less numerous, less active or less effective when we are older. The result is that:

- infections are more likely
- dormant infections can be reactivated
- autoimmune problems, such as rheumatoid arthritis, are more common.

For example, most of the 250,000 cases of pneumonia that happen every year in the UK affect people over 65. Pneumonia is usually caused by an infection. Similarly, most cases of shingles affect older people. Shingles is caused by a flare-up of the virus that causes chickenpox. (A free leaflet on this condition is available from Help the Aged.)

The immune system is able to identify and destroy cancerous cells. The fact that cancer becomes more common as we get older suggests that our ability to identify cancer in its early stages reduces over time.

BOOSTING IMMUNITY

Vaccinations are another effective way of protecting ourselves, in this case against infection. We become more vulnerable to infections as we get older, owing to a decline in the immune system's efficiency. The thymus gland, which plays a key role in building up our immune system when we are young, reaches maximum size at puberty, then begins to shrink. Over time, our circulating lymphocytes, the white cells that attack invading antigens such as viruses, start to lose their responsiveness. So influenza (flu) can be a very serious illness as we get older, with complications such as bronchitis and pneumonia; indeed, it causes thousands of deaths every year in the UK.

People who are eligible for the flu jab every year should take advantage of this service. That means everyone aged 65 and over, as well as younger people in certain at-risk groups, such as those with

JUST A COLD – OR IS IT FLU?

Flu is a virus which first attacks the cells in the respiratory tract. While it can be caught at any time of the year, the most common time is between December and March. Unlike other common viruses, such as chickenpox or measles, there is not just one type of flu virus but many. These types themselves change frequently. This is why getting flu once does not mean that you will not get it again.

The typical symptoms of flu are a high temperature (103°F or 39.4°C) with:

■ chills
■ a cough
■ sore throat
■ general weakness
■ aching muscles in the back, arms or legs.

Often you may also have a headache which might be made worse when you move your eyes.

The major difference between flu and the common cold is that you may be literally 'knocked flat' by flu and unable to do anything but go to bed until the worst of the illness has passed.

The main symptoms of flu generally last for about seven days. However, complications such as bronchitis and pneumonia can delay recovery.

Once the severe illness has passed, you may find that you still feel tired and unwell. This could last for several weeks.

Flu can largely be prevented by vaccination. Vaccines are available through the NHS every year from October, before flu usually strikes. Whereas some vaccines last for years or life, you must get a flu jab every year to stay protected.

chronic asthma, diabetes or chronic liver disease, or who have a lowered immune system due to taking long-term steroid medication.

The vaccine is also offered to people in residential care homes, carers whose charge would be at risk should the carer fall ill, and health-care and social care staff who look after older people, to minimise the possible transmission of influenza to vulnerable patients.

By January 2007, take-up of flu jabs had reached 74 per cent of those aged 65 and over, and 42 per cent of those under 65 in at-risk groups.

The flu vaccine prevents the illness in about three-quarters of those vaccinated. Even if you do catch flu, there is evidence that you will have it more mildly with fewer complications than if you had not been vaccinated. Modern flu vaccines have few side-effects, though some people have a sore arm for a day or two.

Antibiotics are of no use in treating flu. However, they may be used to treat ear or chest infections, which can develop as a result of flu.

TREATMENT OF FLU SYMPTOMS

- Stay in bed and rest as much as you can. This helps your body to fight the infection.
- Drink plenty of non-alcoholic fluids. You need to replace the liquid you lose through sweating.
- Paracetamol, or aspirin and other anti-inflammatory drugs such as ibuprofen can relieve headaches, muscle pains and fever.
- Cough medicines and decongestants can be helpful. But if you are already taking other medications, whether prescribed or bought over the counter, always seek the advice of your pharmacist.
- If you feel very hot and feverish, sponging down with tepid water can reduce body temperature.
- Eat what you can.

SHINGLES

Shingles, which is triggered by the chickenpox virus, causes a painful rash, usually across one side of the body or face. It can only be caught by someone who has already had chickenpox, but there is no obvious reason why the virus becomes active again. The illness is much more common in older people, whose immune systems are becoming weaker with age.

Certain diseases, including cancer and HIV, also make people more susceptible.

Signs of an attack:
- tingling or prickling sensation
- numbness or pain on one side of the body: the pain could be an ache or a shooting/stabbing pain
- high temperature and other flu-like symptoms.

A rash – small groups or bands of blisters – will appear within a few days.

If you think you have shingles, see your GP as soon as possible, because the antiviral drugs that can relieve the pain and shorten the attack (acyclovir, famciclovir or valaciclovir) need to be started within two or three days of the rash appearing.

These drugs will also, if taken in time, ensure that no permanent scars are left by the rash.

People of 65 and older will routinely be offered the pneumo vaccine as well, to protect against pneumonia, septicaemia and bacterial meningitis, caused by *Streptococcus pneumoniae* bacteria. Again, you are also eligible if you are under 65 but suffer from certain diseases, including a heart condition, chronic lung disease, diabetes, a weakened immune system, a damaged spleen or no spleen. Incidentally, the flu and pneumo jabs can be given together.

These, then, are some of the ways in which you can protect yourself from disease, or ensure that it is picked up as early as possible, to improve the chance of cure. So keep up the exercise, watch your weight – and make the most of the years ahead.■

3

KEEPING FIT FOR LIFE

KEEPING FIT FOR LIFE

O f all the things we can do to improve our health, taking exercise leads the field. After we leave school, many of us give up on exercise as a regular, programmed activity, as we take on the pressures of adult life. If that is what happened in your case, it might be time to re-consider.

THE CASE FOR EXERCISE

If there is an 'elixir of youth', exercise is it. We all know that it's good for us, but many of us are only paying lip service to the idea. Few of us realise just how much exercise helps our health once we get to middle age and beyond.

One of the most dangerous ideas around is that retirement should be a time of 'slowing down' and 'putting our feet up'. The truth is that in the UK every 15 minutes someone dies as a direct result of physical inactivity. Relaxation is important but we also need regular exercise to stay active, healthy and independent. And just 30 minutes a day of any activity that makes you slightly breathless or feeling warmer will help stave off heart disease and other illnesses.

It is not that the exercise message is not being heard, but even though three out of five 50–65-year-olds know what the recommended amount of exercise is, many still choose to shun the health advice. In fact, only 30 per cent of 50–64-year-olds in the UK take the recommended amount of physical activity, and for 65–84-year-olds this dwindles to 6 per cent.

Meanwhile, a recent poll has shown that nearly 60 per cent of over-50s are concerned that they are not getting enough exercise. Many (62 per cent) are not interested in joining a gym. Over half are put off by the cost of joining, while 60 per cent say gyms do not offer the type of exercise they are interested in. Only 24 per cent are happy with the aerobics/dance facilities provided by their local authority, and only 31 per cent are happy with the racquet sports facilities. Most (58 per cent) do not know what dance/aer-obics facilities are provided by their local authorities. In fact, all local authorities have a list of activities they provide for the over-50s in their area.

Now a drive is under way that should make it easier to enjoy the sort of exercise you feel drawn to, and to find instructors who have appropriate training and are sensitive to the needs and concerns of the over-50s. Already, exercise is known to be so important for good health that GPs and hospital specialists can prescribe it through an exercise referral system, or you can ask your local health authority about it. You are given a personal programme for classes at your local leisure or sports centre, or you can join a local exercise, walking or swimming group. However, although growing, the system across the country is patchy.

The National Coalition for Active Ageing is now urging fitness and recreation providers to partner with the medical community to create a nationwide network of such schemes, and to provide exercise sessions which are culturally appropriate, such as running ethnic dance classes where modest dress is the norm, with bilingual instructors. It is also encouraging schools to open up their facilities to community use, so that people over 50 can participate in physical activity programmes.

If the gym does not appeal, there are plenty of simple and cheap alternative ways to exercise. Try thinking of everyday activities as a way of getting fit.

- Just walking up and down stairs for five minutes a day will keep your legs in good shape and help maintain bone density; 10 minutes a day will burn off 100 calories.
- Use stairs instead of lifts and escalators whenever possible.
- Park the car at a distance from your destination, get off the bus or Tube a couple of stops early, and walk the rest.
- Hold a couple of cans of soup when doing arm lifts and

stretches, and graduate to two-litre bottles of water as you get stronger.

- Always bend at the knees when lifting things, so that you do not injure your back.

If you find a task challenging, practise until you get better at it: this is the best way to train the body.

Gardening is great exercise, but do some stretches first to warm up, and take a bath (not a shower) afterwards, to get rid of any stiffness you may feel.

If you enjoy the outdoors, consider joining the Green Gym scheme run by BTCV. It is free of charge, and might even be prescribed by your GP. Groups meet in their local area at least once a week for a session of up to three hours, to engage on environmental conservation or gardening activities with a trained leader. Sessions open and close with basic warm-up exercises and cool-down activities.

Outdoor activity in a green environment boosts mental well-being, too.

In a comparison study 20 people suffering from mental health illnesses were allocated either a 30-minute walk in a country park or a walk in an indoor shopping centre. After the country walk, 71 per cent reported decreased levels of depression, while 90 per cent reported increased self-esteem. This contrasted with only 45 per cent who experienced a decrease in depression after the shopping centre walk, with 22 per cent even saying they actually felt more depressed. In a separate study, 94 per cent of participants said green activities had benefited their mental health and lifted their depression, while 90 per cent said the combination of nature and exercise had the greatest effect.

THE HEART OF THE MATTER

Medical scientists from many different disciplines, from sports medicine to orthopaedics to immunology, have proved that every function needs exercise to keep it running at its peak.

First of all, exercise benefits the heart by making it stronger, thus reducing the risk of coronary heart disease. Arteries benefit by becoming more elastic, expanding and letting more blood through. Moreover, exercise reduces the risk of blood clots and clogged-up arteries (atherosclerosis). Blood pressure can be kept under control by exercise. High blood pressure is a major risk factor for heart disease, stroke and other serious illnesses. With better blood circulation, there is less of a tendency to get swollen ankles (oedema) or to feel cold at the extremities.

When our heart and arteries (cardiovascular system) are working efficiently they are making oxygen and nutrients available to muscles, bone and brain cells, where they have important jobs to do. Significantly, people who exercise regularly have more energy and are more alert than those who are sedentary. Exercise also decreases the risk of glaucoma and the craving for nicotine.

STAYING STRONG

Exercise is vital to maintain muscle strength and bone density, both of which decline naturally as we age.

Muscle strength is vital to perform daily activities such as getting out of the bath or a chair. With inactivity, muscle quickly wastes away; after only two weeks in bed recovering from, say, flu, we can lose 1–2 per cent of bone density and up to 20 per cent of our strength. Muscle weakness round the major joints can lead to osteoarthritis, a painful condition affecting the cartilage and bone around the joints.

Thinning bones – osteoporosis – is a major cause of fractures in the wrist, hip and spine. Exercise stimulates the production of growth hormone which helps to maintain muscle and bone. Outdoor exercise tops up levels of vitamin D (from sunshine), which is also vital for bone health. People who have a condition such as osteoarthritis can eliminate the pain this brings by building muscle strength around the affected joint. Exercise can prevent falls, a major threat to people in the oldest age groups.

Exercise helps to regulate our metabolism (all the chemical and physical processes that enable us to function), controlling our weight and reducing the risk of Type 2 diabetes, while many who have this form of diabetes can keep it under control with regular exercise and diet.

Our immune system benefits enormously from exercise, although exactly how is not fully understood. An efficient immune system doesn't just ward off colds and flu. Scientists now believe that exercise can lower our risk of many cancers, including cancers of the colon, breast, uterus, ovaries, prostate gland, testes and lung (even in smokers).

PUTTING THE SPARKLE IN LIFE

Exercise helps to keep our brains healthy. Only four arteries supply blood to the brain so arterial health and avoiding blood clots is vital to prevent strokes and vascular dementia and even preserve our memories and understanding.

Exercise improves our mood by releasing endorphins from the brain – in fact, the 'feel-good' factor is the reason why regular exercisers can't give it up. Stress, anxiety and some types of depression can be helped by exercise, which also improves the duration and quality of sleep. Exercise can also bring many social benefits, such as new friendships and fun, which in turn improve well-being.

Immobility is highly dangerous as we get older. As well as all the risks listed above, immobility can lead to incontinence, constipation, poor wound-healing and risk of leg ulcers, deep vein thrombosis, pressure sores and oedema (ankle swelling) – all unnecessary side-effects of sedentary behaviour.

THE CASE AGAINST EXERCISE

We do not know of any case against exercise. If we exercise carefully, doing exercise that is correctly targeted and paced, there are no known harmful side-effects. Some people need to be careful about what exercise they do and how they do it, including those with heart disease, osteoporosis, arthritis and asthma. Even so, everyone can do some form of exercise and it will help improve each of these conditions if carefully managed.

If you are concerned, it is best to exercise in a group with an instructor who is qualified to adapt exercise to suit any medical condition and to ensure safety and effectiveness. Always talk to your own doctor before you start any unaccustomed exercise, to check what is safe for you.

Convinced yet? We know that we are never too old to start exercising or to do a bit more. Research shows that we will benefit if we become more active more often, whatever our age – it is never too late.

EXERCISE: ARE YOU KIDDING?

In later life we need the right strategies to keep us active and fit, but that doesn't mean workouts from dawn till dusk. A major problem is that we confuse lack of fitness for the signs of 'getting on' and adopt the wrong strategies. For example, when going upstairs becomes uncomfortable, we take the lift or move to a bungalow, depriving ourselves of the benefits of that exercise. Limiting the exercise we take is the first step on the slippery slope that leads to dependency and ill-health. Twenty-first century living does not help, of course: the car and the remote control, for example, limit our everyday exercise.

We cannot store the benefits of exercise, unfortunately. If you were sporty until your 40s, it will not help in your 70s (except that you may have a higher baseline to lose strength from).

WHAT KIND OF EXERCISE DO WE NEED?

If it is to be beneficial we need exercise to maintain, or ideally improve:

- strength
- bone density
- stamina
- power
- balance
- flexibility.

Strength is the muscle power to perform everyday tasks such as walking, climbing stairs, lifting and, ultimately, getting out of the bath or a chair and even breathing efficiently. Loss of muscle strength alone will lead to disability and loss of independence. Women are particularly vulnerable because they have less muscle mass to begin with and so lose strength more quickly. Nearly 50 per cent of older women do not have enough strength in their legs to rise from a chair without also using their arms to push.

Without appropriate exercise the next stage is to be stuck in the chair until someone hauls us out. It is vital to maintain strength in the main functional muscles – the legs, arms, ankles and back.

You can improve strength by holding a movement for a slow count of five and repeating it on a regular basis. For example, while washing up, strengthen your ankles by rising on to your toes and holding it for a count of five, then gently lower yourself and repeat it.

Bone density Loss of bone makes fractures more likely and can cause the upper spine to collapse, which in turn makes breathing difficult. When bone thins to a certain degree, we call it osteoporosis, which you can read more about on pages 143–6. Bone density can be maintained only by weight-bearing exercise: it is the stress on bone and the jarring repetition of movement that builds bone mineral density. We particularly need to maintain bone at three sites – the wrist, hip and spine. Squeezing a tennis ball 10 times a day, holding each squeeze for five seconds, will help improve bone density at the wrist within six months. Joining a keep-fit class that includes lots of standing work and strength work will help maintain or improve bone density at the hip and spine.

Stamina or **cardiovascular fitness** is vital to ensure that the heart and arteries are supplying energy-giving oxygen to all the cells and to help keep the whole system free from disease. Any exercise that makes you warm and increases your rate of breathing (also called aerobic exercise) will benefit your cardiovascular system. We need stamina to avoid undue tiredness, which is often attributed to medical conditions rather than unfitness. However, the benefits occur only if the activity is maintained for at least half an hour (though this can be split into short bursts of 10 or 15 minutes during a day) and on a regular basis – three times a week or more.

Power is the ability to use our muscles fast when we need them. For example, to prevent a trip from becoming a fall we must be able to correct a trip quickly. We lose our power more quickly than our strength as it is not only the performance of the muscle that is important but also the nervous system's ability to receive and send information between the muscle and brain. Power can be improved by both strength and endurance (cardiovascular fitness) work. It is also important to maintain co-ordination and reaction time, perhaps through ball games or dance routines.

Balance ensures we stay upright at all times. Loss of balance predisposes us to falls and hence fractures. Balance is maintained by the integration of our nervous system and our muscular system – vision, inner ear balance and feedback from receptors in muscles and joints all contribute to the feedback mechanisms that we need to stay upright. Good co-ordination, strength, power and balance are vital to prevent a trip from becoming a fall. You can read more about falls on pages 53–5.

Flexibility ensures that we can perform a range of movements needed for everyday tasks: for example, bending to tie shoelaces, or stretching to change a light bulb. Nearly a quarter of those over 50 do not have adequate shoulder flexibility to wash their hair or do up zips behind their back. Flexibility of the spine, in particular, needs to be maintained if we want to avoid stiffness and back pain. Indeed, stiffness in the joints is one of the reasons why some reactions slow down in later life.

Moving the joints around reduces stiffness, so try to stretch and rotate all of them through the fullest range of movement twice a day, especially after getting up in the morning. This needs to be done carefully, so if you are not sure about it join an exercise class.

However, **no single form of exercise delivers all these benefits**. Walking, for example, which we all know to be healthy, does little for balance or flexibility. Swimming does nothing for bone density because the water is taking our weight. Yoga does little for the cardiovascular system. This is why we need to 'pick and mix' types of exercise to get a broad range of benefits.

HOW MUCH EXERCISE DO WE NEED?

- Half-hour blocks of exercise once or twice a week will maintain our independence.
- Two-and-a-half hours of moderate exercise a week will keep us in the best of health.

How much exercise we need depends on our goals, but what is

astonishing, given all the benefits that exercise brings, is not how much we need, but how little. If the goal is simply to maintain independence, half-hour blocks of exercise once or twice a week, which can be carried out as 10- or 15-minute bouts during a day, will prevent us crumbling into dependency, according to scientists' current understanding.

However, we all need at least an hour a day of pottering about in our own homes and gardens, and ideally walking to the shops, to maintain a basic level of fitness. There is more exercise value than we realise in being on our feet (which helps to prevent bone loss), going up and down stairs and lifting (this maintains strength), doing housework, gardening and DIY (which help balance, flexibility, cardiovascular fitness).

If the goal is to maintain exuberant good health, scientists are confident that we can achieve it with just two-and-a-half hours of moderate exercise each week in addition to daily routines.

'Moderate exercise' is exercise that makes us warm and slightly breathless and which is progressive: that is, it challenges us to do a bit more each time. We do not need to take this exercise all in one go, but we do need blocks of at least half an hour to get the maximum benefit. So five half-hour sessions per week would be enough. There are 112 waking hours in a week, so two-and-a half hours is a very small investment for a phenomenal return.

The important thing is to do what you can: any exercise is better than none at all. Put simply, we should aim to be more active, more often.

SURELY NOT AT OUR AGE?

Just two-and-a-half hours a week of appropriate exercise will keep us in the prime of health: a small investment for a huge return.

Although exercise can be risky if it is inappropriate or badly taught, we cannot say it loud enough: science tells us that we are never too old to benefit from some form of exercise. No health condition rules out some form of exercise and even people who are completely chair-bound can improve their health and well-being with tailored exercise.

However, if you are very athletic take care not to over-exercise. Older muscle is less efficient at repairing itself and damaged muscles take much longer to recover. By far the most damaging form of exercise is running downhill, when the muscles are used as brakes: unless you have done this most of your life, avoid running down mountains or very steep hills. Even walking down a steep hill should be done carefully. If you are heading for the hills and are unused to them, build up muscle strength gradually by brisk walking on the flat first.

In the next few pages we list some popular forms of exercise and explain what science now tells us about their benefits.

TRY THESE FOR SIZE . . .

It is really important to find types of exercise that we enjoy. We need to do more than one kind to get the full range of benefits. Here are some popular choices with details of what science tells us they can offer.

Walking/rambling has to be brisk (making you mildly breathless if you try to talk at the same time) to bring any benefit at all. A stroll won't help. Walking/rambling:

- is good for stamina and cardiovascular fitness
- maintains muscle strength in the legs, and
- helps prevent bone loss.

However, it does not help general flexibility or balance.
Verdict Good leg muscles are vital for getting the blood back up the

legs to the heart, so walking should ideally be part of every older person's routine. Running produces similar benefits but is particularly beneficial for cardiovascular fitness and bone health.

Swimming also has to be 'brisk' to bring real benefit. It can:

- develop muscle strength
- improve cardiovascular fitness
- boost flexibility – for example, in the shoulders – and
- deliver benefits for people who cannot bear their own weight.

Aquaerobics (exercises done standing in water) can help to maintain balance. But swimming does nothing for bone density and can cause neck problems.
Verdict Probably over-rated and needs to complemented by weight-bearing exercise for older people.

Cycling (whether in the open air or on an exercise bike) is excellent for:

- cardiovascular health
- lower body strength and power
- balance (only if using a bike that moves)
- ankle and foot flexibility.

Verdict A great form of exercise, though it does not maintain bone and a stationary exercise bike will not help balance.

Tennis and badminton are terrific ways of maintaining:

- cardiovascular fitness
- speed and stamina

- muscle tone and power
- bone in the preferred arm (but be careful not to put it under too much strain)
- balance
- flexibility, to some extent.

Verdict First-rate, but if you have not played in ages you must approach these gently and do them regularly. An occasional game may do more harm than good.

Keep-fit/aerobics in a structured class programme can bring all the benefits of all types of exercise, but it depends on what is covered. A gentle, seated exercise class may be fun but may not be effective. Ensure your teacher is qualified. Exercise books and videos can be helpful too, but they do not encourage progression. Canadian Air Force exercises are not recommended for anyone past 55: some of the exercises are now known to be dangerous.

Verdict Warmly recommended but make sure your instructor is qualified to instruct older people. (Extend is the organisation that can help: see chapter 10. Alternatively, be sure to pick a seniors-qualified exercise instructor, contactable through the YMCA or the Keep Fit Association, for example.)

Yoga/pilates have not been rigorously studied by scientists but the consensus is that they:

- maintain flexibility
- maintain muscle tone and strength
- reduce anxiety
- develop body awareness.

The latter is important because, as we age, the sensors that tell us where the body parts are become less efficient. There is more about

this on pages 53–5, where we discuss the prevention of falls.
Verdict In scientific terms, not proven, but do not let that stop you.

T'ai chi has undergone much research. A Chinese invention, *t'ai chi* is a slow, highly choreographed programme of exercise movements that:

- develop strength
- boost flexibility
- improve body awareness
- improve balance (above all)
- reduce anxiety and stress.

Verdict An excellent form of exercise for older people, but add something for cardiovascular health.

Golf can develop bone density in the preferred arm, and the concentration required in focusing on the ball will take your mind off any worries. But otherwise it is often too leisurely to be of much benefit.
Verdict The main benefit is social, but that is important too.

Dance can be beneficial for:

- balance
- flexibility
- cardiovascular fitness
- power
- co-ordination and
- reaction.

Verdict It depends what you do and how energetically. The balance, co-ordination and social benefits are first-rate.

Gym exercise mainly benefits our:

- strength and
- cardiovascular system.

Gyms also offer support from professionals, but check that they are trained to work with older adults. Many gyms now offer sessions for mature people so we do not feel out of place.

Verdict Highly effective but often expensive, especially if you do not attend regularly.

Sex is exercise too, though it depends what we do and for how long. Energetic sex can support cardiovascular fitness and, ladies, splaying the legs exercises the muscles you need to get into and out of the bath. And because it releases feel-good endorphins from the brain, you could find yourself going around with a big smile on your face for some time afterwards.

Verdict Limited as a form of exercise but highly recommended; people with a healthy sex life do appear to have a health advantage.

Walking the dog

A dog is many things – a reason to take exercise, a confidence booster when you are out, a companion, and a source of much entertainment. But it is easy to believe that because we walk the dog, we are getting useful exercise. Too many people, unfortunately, stroll rather than walk the dog. Both you and the dog need brisk walks that build up in length and challenges as you progress. For example, when walking a mile on the flat gets to be easy, add on an extra half-mile or walk uphill. Both you and the dog will be rejuvenated.

IF YOU ARE UNWELL ...

Exercising when you are unwell, particularly if you have a significant infection, may damage your muscles. But do not immobilise yourself

EXERCISE TIPS

- Build physical activity into your daily routine.
- Walk a bit more briskly and use the stairs more often.
- Start any new activity with care and progress slowly.
- Aim to become involved in physical activity at least three times a week for at least 20 minutes.
- Wear loose clothing and soft-soled shoes.
- Always warm up first to avoid injury to muscles and slow down gradually before you stop.
- Set yourself realistic and achievable goals.
- Join a class or exercise with friends: it makes exercise that much more enjoyable and should mean you are less likely to give up.
- Don't hold your breath while doing any movement.
- Don't exercise if you are tired, unwell or have just eaten.
- Don't turn your head or look up at the ceiling quickly as such movements can cause dizziness.
- Unless you really want to, don't buy special equipment for exercising at home. Instead, use bags of flour or sugar (wrapped well in case they split) or tin cans as weights, and pairs of tights to provide resistance.

during illness: it is vital to keep moving about to avoid the risk of thrombosis and muscle-wasting. Gentle pottering in your own home is the most you should attempt until you are fully recovered.

TAKE CARE NOT TO FALL

A third of people over the age of 65 have a fall at least once a year. Falls can be catastrophic: they are the main cause of injury leading to hospital admission or death for people aged over 65. Half of those who break a hip never recover independent mobility. But there is nothing inevitable about falls: to a large extent they can be prevented by suitable exercise.

There are specific exercises you can do to improve your strength and balance, which everyone can benefit from improving. Exercises to strengthen the muscles of your legs and body and to improve co-ordination and balance are known as 'balance training'. As well as increasing general fitness, balance training is one of the most effective ways to reduce the risk of falling.

Balance training is especially important if you have problems resulting from illness, such as joint pain, weakness or feeling dizzy or unsteady. Balance training can help you get back to normal and overcome feelings of stiffness or unsteadiness. If you have difficulty getting around, it can make it easier for you to get out and about without needing support or someone with you all the time.

You can fit balance training into your daily life by carrying out simple exercises at home as and when it suits you. Alternatively, you may prefer to join a group at a local centre, where a professional can advise you. This will also give you the opportunity to get to know people, learn from others, and use special training equipment or play sports. To find out about balance training classes in your local area, ask at your local library, health centre, leisure centre or Age Concern group.

As with any exercise, take it gently at first and build up slowly.

Always begin with a warm-up to prepare your body and finish by cooling-down. If you're not used to taking physical exercise, speak to your doctor first. If you experience chest pain or feel faint you should stop exercising and contact your doctor.

Most people find that balance training is easier than they expected – and more enjoyable. You may be surprised by how much you can achieve.

You can talk to your doctor about how to get the most out of strength and balance training. You will benefit most from an exercise programme specially designed to meet your needs. This is especially important if you have had a fall or are at all unsteady on your feet. Don't give up on exercising just because you have had a fall or are afraid of falling. Reducing your physical activity can actually make you *more* prone to falling.

A BALANCING ACT

There are 200 documented risk factors for falls, ranging from the drowsiness brought on by some medications and alcohol to wearing bifocals. But our trips may become falls if our balance is impaired, muscles weak and reactions slow, so that we cannot get a leg out fast enough to stabilise ourselves.

Balance is a complex business involving the brain, inner-ear mechanisms, information from the eyes and ears, sensors in the body which tell us where we are, motor nerves and joints. However, balance can be trained: we do not need to lose it as we age. We can also improve general fitness, which will speed up reaction times and give us enough leg strength to cope if we trip.

The previous pages showed that relatively few types of exercise actually help our balance, so it pays to choose carefully, or to go to a class specifically targeted at older fallers. One exercise to consider is *t'ai chi*. Practitioners suggest this gentle exercise system can reduce the risk of falling by 47 per cent. However, if you are already falling and are not too confident of your balance, you must go for an assessment with your GP to find out why. You may need a specially tailored class as general *t'ai chi* won't meet your needs. See page 53 for how to find out about balance training exercises in your area.

FEET: TAKING CARE OF THE FOUNDATIONS

Our feet and ankles hold up the entire edifice of our body, yet we rarely consider their need for exercise. Staying upright and balanced depends heavily on having strong foot and ankle muscles, flexibility and effective sensors.

About half of our body sensors are in our feet, but because we wear shoes they become desensitised. One reason we fall when we are older is that we do not know with complete accuracy where our feet are, and do not raise our feet enough to get over obstacles.

Take care of your feet by targeting them with specific exercise to keep the muscles strong and joints and tendons flexible. Many yoga classes cover this and, because yoga is done in bare feet, it retrains the foot sensors. Swollen feet and ankles (oedema) will restrict movement and if you suffer from this you need an exercise such as brisk walking to get the blood circulating, then rest with your feet up.

To ensure we can care for our feet and cut our own toenails, we need to work on our flexibility, particularly of the spine. Yoga, *t'ai chi*, some keep-fit exercises, and even gardening and housework are all good for maintaining flexibility.

TIME TO RELAX

Rest and sleep are vital for health and well-being, but how much rest do we need and what should we do if sleep eludes us or is not refreshing?

REST AND RELAXATION

We all think we know when we need to rest because we are tired. Particularly after exercising, rest is important: you should never exercise to the point of exhaustion. We need plenty of rest when recovering from illness. But many people become tired after doing nothing much at all.

If that describes you, you should see your doctor to rule out underlying conditions such as anaemia or thyroid problems. (In the UK, sleep disorders represent the biggest single reason why people over 65 contact their GP; women are 30 per cent more likely than men to report insomnia.) But you may simply need more exercise, because without it you are not getting enough oxygen, so you feel sluggish and tired all the time. In later life we tend to do too little. Rest should occupy an occasional weekend, not 20 years of your life.

When we do rest, we can give it added value by learning a relaxation technique. Scientists now know that relaxation methods such as yoga, t'ai chi, meditation and prayer help to lower blood pressure, produce alpha waves in the brain (the mental state of relaxation), slow the heart and breathing and even enhance the immune system. This kind of deep relaxation is especially helpful for dealing with stress and anxiety.

A GOOD NIGHT'S SLEEP

Lack of sleep – or sleeping at the wrong time – really matters to our quality of life and our health. According to US researchers, sleeping for at least four to seven hours a night even helps us to live longer. We appear to need the same amount of sleep throughout our adult lives, but scientists have confirmed that sleep patterns tend to change as we age, with sleep being more broken; it is not clear why this happens.

Typically, older people wake more frequently during the night, experience more day-time tiredness and consequently take naps during the day. Some people become sleepier early in the evening, and wake earlier in the morning.

One of the most marked changes that occurs with age is that stage IV sleep, the phase of 'deep' and restorative sleep, declines, and is sometimes even absent. Part of the problem is that if people are waking more frequently, it takes longer for them to cycle through the various stages of sleep to reach stage IV.

Lack of sleep has wide-reaching consequences. People with insomnia are four times more likely to suffer from depression than people who sleep well. Safety – both at home and on the road – can be affected by sleepiness, and after a poor night's sleep many people report accomplishing fewer daily tasks and enjoying activities less. Memory and mental performance are also adversely affected. Many older people can find themselves too tired to undertake social activities with family and friends, which leads to increasing isolation.

No matter what your age, getting the proper amount of restorative sleep remains essential to your physical health and emotional well-being. There is mounting evidence that poor sleep can lead to serious diseases that affect the quality of life. Research has suggested that sleep loss can impair immune function, possibly hindering the ability of older people to fight off illness.

It is during sleep when natural killer cells (part of the body's defence mechanism against viruses, bacteria and even cancer) are generated. A study at the Cerrahpasa Medical School in Turkey found that after 24 hours of sleep deprivation the percentage of natural killer cells in the blood declined by 37 per cent. A study from the University of California, San Diego, found that one night of partial sleep deprivation reduced natural-killer-cell activity to 72 per cent of normal levels.

Data from the Nurses' Health Study, an ongoing study including more than 78,000 women, found that at the ten-year stage women who worked between one and 29 years on a rotating night-shift schedule (and hence suffered problems with sleep) had an 8 per cent increase in breast cancer risk, which might be partly explained by weakened immune systems.

Simple measures can improve the quality of our sleep. A good daily sleep/wake routine is all-important. Do not go to bed until you feel you cannot stay awake, but always get up at the same time each day, including weekends. Exposure to the sun is invaluable for setting your body clock, so try to get outdoors each day.

If you are having trouble sleeping, in the four hours before bed-time avoid heavy meals, alcohol (it helps you doze off but disrupts your sleep pattern), tea, coffee and stimulating activities; also avoid late-night exercise, as it might boost your energy levels. If you wake up in the small hours, get up and do something dull, like cleaning shoes. Write down your thoughts to deal with later if you wake with your mind racing. The text box opposite contains more tips for improving sleep.

If you feel sleepy after lunch, have a short nap (up to an hour) but never nap after about 5pm as this will prevent you sleeping at night. And get some exercise: nothing improves sleep so much as being healthily tired. ∎

TIPS FOR IMPROVING YOUR SLEEP

People all too often accept sleep difficulties as a natural part of ageing, not realising that lifestyle changes can be easily introduced to improve quality of sleep.

Try these suggestions, and if they don't work see your GP to rule out whether there are any underlying health problems preventing you from sleeping.

Consider keeping a sleep diary where you record information for a few weeks on when you go to bed, how often you wake, and when you nap during the day to give your GP a clear picture of your sleep patterns.

- Make sure your room is quiet and dark and your bed comfortable. Avoid activities such as writing letters in bed.
- Get up and go to bed at the same time every day. If you must take a nap during the day, limit yourself to an hour.
- Develop a relaxing pre-sleep ritual: for example, having a bath or drinking a glass of warm milk or herbal tea.
- Don't toss and turn for longer than 20 minutes. If you can't sleep, get up and do something calming, such as reading.
- Limit your caffeine and alcohol use, and eat dinner at least two to three hours before bedtime. It's more difficult to fall asleep if your body is still breaking down food.
- Give up smoking. Nicotine is a stimulant and when smokers go to sleep they experience nicotine withdrawal.
- Exercise regularly. Physical activity early in the day may promote deeper, better-quality sleep. Too-vigorous exercise just before bedtime, however, may delay sleep.
- Make sure you're spending enough time outdoors. Sunlight helps the body's circadian rhythm to work appropriately and gauge when to sleep.

4

EATING
FOR
HEALTH

EATING FOR HEALTH

The link between a good diet and staying healthy is well known. But few of us are aware that our nutritional needs change as we age. Although scientists are still some way from understanding exactly what makes an optimum diet for older people, they can tell us which particular nutrients and what style of diet are vital to maintain health and independence.

WHY DIET MATTERS

Nutrition is now a science in its own right but many other disciplines are contributing to our understanding of how diet shapes our health. Every process in our bodies, from repair and maintenance of cells to the complex operation of, say, the immune system requires a specific mix of proteins, carbohydrates, fats, vitamins, minerals, trace elements and water to make it function. Dozens of nutrients are involved and their relationship with each other is often critical. For example, it is impossible to use the calcium in our diets without vitamin D to help process it, while vitamin C makes it easier for the body to absorb iron.

Take eye health. Diet has been shown to be linked to cataract and age-related macular degeneration (AMD), the biggest cause of vision loss among older people. Bone health is highly dependent on good diet, as is our cardiovascular system. Our arteries can become clogged with 'bad' cholesterol (low-density lipoproteins or LDL) as a result of eating too much saturated fat, while other nutrients offer protection. Blood itself needs adequate iron, vitamin B12 and folic acid, without which we become vulnerable to anaemia.

A healthy immune system depends on adequate intakes of vitamin C, zinc and other nutrients. Poor wound-healing may be the result of zinc deficiency. Diet is thought to be linked to about one-third of all cancers, including those of the lung, stomach, oesophagus, colon and breast. Degenerative disorders such as Parkinson's disease are linked in part to oxidative damage, linked with free radical production, which in turn may be prevented to some extent by diet. Depression can be caused by lack of B vitamins.

Obesity is the biggest nutritional disorder in the developed world and is especially common in middle-aged and older people. It increases the risk of coronary heart disease, stroke, Type 2 diabetes, osteoarthritis, colon and breast cancer.

Few of us need convincing that a good diet is a sound principle, but we can delude ourselves that because we have reached a reasonable age, we must be getting it right. We can all make improvements to our diet and it is never too late to make changes that will bring benefits, as the next few pages show.

A GOOD DIET FOR OVER-55s

Dietary advice has changed little in the past 30 years but scientists are now beginning to establish our special needs as we get older. Some of them may surprise you.

ADDED NUTRITION FOR ADDED YEARS

Scientists are clear about one thing – we need a better diet as we get older. Our calorie requirements become slightly lower as we age because we are less active, but the need for nutrients stays the same or may even increase. In other words, smaller servings of food need to be 'nutritionally dense' to provide all we need from it. It is difficult for scientists to make specific recommendations because the way we digest, absorb, use and excrete nutrients not only changes as we age, it also varies widely between individuals.

For example, our liver shrinks in size over time and becomes less metabolically active, which reduces its ability to process potentially toxic substances, including medicines and alcohol – drug dose levels may need to be reduced in older people, and women, in particular, may find that they cannot handle alcohol as they once did.

In simple terms, however, we should be eating:

- plenty of food that packs a nutritional punch, such as fruit and vegetables, wholewheat bread and other cereals, fish and meat (or vegetarian alternatives including pulses), milk and dairy foods. These are the basics and we need to eat some of these food groups every day; and
- fewer 'treat' foods such as sugar, cakes, biscuits, sweets and chocolate bars, sugary drinks, crisps and other nibbles. It is best to regard all of these as an occasional treat.

This 'senior diet', by the way, is also one that helps to keep our weight in check.

We need variety in our food as we age. This is not just to spice up our lives – though that's important, too – but because research has shown that older people who have a monotonous diet or who exclude whole food groups are at risk of missing out key nutrients. People at risk include vegans, people who do not eat any fruit or vegetables, or dairy produce, some vegetarians, and those who know what day of the week it is from what is on the menu. We need to eat as many types of food as possible.

THE ANTI-AGEING REMEDY: FRUIT AND VEGETABLES

'Eat at least five portions of fruit and vegetables a day' has long been the advice from the government. And it looks as though the message is starting to get through. Research from Nielson is showing that since 2005 sales of so-called 'superfoods' have shot up. Beans, blueberries, broccoli, oats, oranges, pumpkin, salmon, soya, spinach, green or black tea, tomatoes, turkey, walnuts and yoghurt have shown massive sales growth.

So what is so special about fruit and vegetables? The vitamins and minerals they contain have a wide range of jobs to do, not least of which is mopping up damaging free radicals, a common culprit in age-related disorders.

Oxygen, though vital for life, comes with a high price-tag. Oxygen is a highly reactive element which, in the body, combines with other molecules to form free radicals – high-energy chemical substances which seek out something to combine with.

Free radicals are, frankly, scary. They will attack cell membranes, proteins and even DNA, causing irreversible damage. Many degenerative diseases that are common in later life are likely to be exacerbated, and in some instances may actually be caused, by free radical damage: cancer, vascular diseases, degenerative eye diseases and possibly neuro-degenerative diseases such as Parkinson's. There are other sources of 'oxidative stress', including tobacco smoke, other pollutants, certain drugs and excess alcohol.

Luckily for us, there is one way to lock up free radicals before they do much damage – through the anti-oxidant vitamins and minerals found in fruit and vegetables. The main anti-oxidant vitamins are carotenoids and vitamins A, C and E, while key minerals are zinc, copper, manganese and selenium. Carotenoids are particularly powerful antioxidants; they include beta-carotene (found in carrots), lycopene, lutein and zeaxanthine.

We have other anti-oxidant defences, such as natural enzymes, but scientists have established that we need to consume anti-oxidants in large, regular doses – hence the advice about five portions of fruit and vegetables every day. Smokers use antioxidants faster and therefore need an even higher intake.

Different fruits and vegetables offer different protection. For example, green leafy vegetables and vitamin C-rich fruits and vegetables offer the greatest protection against heart disease. Eating foods rich in lutein – such as sweetcorn, spinach, courgettes, green peppers, cucumbers, red grapes and kiwis – may protect against cataract and macular degeneration, as may zeaxanthine, which comes from everything orange – peppers, corn, oranges and mangoes. Lycopene appears to protect against heart disease and prostate cancer, and a particularly rich source is tomatoes – if they are cooked. So you really can enjoy tomato ketchup and tomato sauces knowing they are health foods.

As we cannot know what scientists will reveal next about the way free radicals work and which foodstuffs hold them in check, it is a good insurance policy to eat a wide variety of fruit and vegetables. Fruit and vegetables have many other important jobs to do, including lowering our blood pressure, because the potassium they contain increases sodium (salt) excretion. Potassium is found in many fruits and vegetables including bananas, citrus fruits, raisins and other dried fruits, potatoes and avocados.

WHAT DOES 'FIVE PORTIONS' MEAN?

'Five portions' does not mean five helpings of fruit and five of vegetables, simply five portions of either. If you are unsure what a portion is, see below.

Fruit

Apple, orange or banana = 1 fruit
Very large fruit (e.g. melon or pineapple) = 1 large slice
Small fruits (e.g. plums, kiwis, satsumas) = 2 fruits
Raspberries, strawberries and grapes = 1 cupful
Fresh fruit salad or stewed or canned fruit = 2–3 tablespoons
Dried fruit = $1/2$–1 tablespoon
Fruit juice = 1 glass (150ml). (Note that drinking more than one glass does not count as a second portion of fruit.)

Vegetables

Raw, cooked, frozen or canned vegetables = 2 tablespoons
Salad = 1 dessert bowl

Fresh vegetables and fruit are the 'best buy' nutritionally, but frozen, canned and dried produce counts too. Potatoes do not count as a vegetable but are a good source of carbohydrate and fibre if you eat the skin, so do not stop eating them.

If you cannot eat five portions of fruit and vegetables a day, eat what you can – every little helps. Start now – it's never too late.

If you do not like fruit and vegetables at all, try new ways of cooking them; not many people would find boiled cabbage and carrots exciting, but you could try stir-frying instead. Stir-frying is quick, tasty and retains the nutrients well. Many vegetables can be roasted – try carrots, peppers, courgettes, even cauliflower and broccoli – preferably in olive oil. Raw vegetables such as grated carrots or courgettes can give added interest to salads or sandwiches. You can 'disguise' vegetables in casseroles and liquidised soups, and the fruit in pies and puddings is still fruit.

If all else fails, take a suitable vitamin supplement but remember that pills do not match the real thing and will not provide fibre.

FOOD CHECKLIST
Eating well means enjoying your food and having plenty of variety. These are the foods you should try to eat each day.

Fruit and vegetables
Try to eat a variety of fruit, vegetables and salads. They are full of vitamins, antioxidants, minerals and fibre. Aim to eat five portions a day. Frozen, canned or dried fruit and vegetables, and fruit juice, are just as good for you as fresh produce. Use fruit and vegetables that are canned in water or their natural juice rather than syrup or oil. Try to include some fruit and vegetables at each meal and have fruit as a snack between meals.

Meat, poultry, fish, eggs, beans, lentils and nuts
Eat a portion of any of these foods at two of your meals each day. All these foods contain proteins which build and repair your body. You do not need to eat meat or fish every day – cheese, well-cooked eggs, beans or lentils can be eaten instead.

Foods containing fat and sugar

Sugary and fatty foods provide energy and can make meals taste better, but use them sparingly if you are watching your weight as they are high in calories. Don't eat these foods at the expense of other, more nutritious, foods.

Bread, other cereals and potatoes

Try to have a serving of starchy food (such as bread, breakfast cereal, potatoes, rice, noodles or pasta) with every meal. These foods give energy. Wholegrain cereals have more B vitamins, minerals and fibre, which keep us well and help prevent constipation.

Milk and dairy foods

These foods contain calcium which helps to keep bones strong. Try to have three servings a day. A serving can be:

- 1 cup of milk
- 1 yoghurt or fromage frais
- 25g (1oz) cheese
- a small pot of cottage cheese
- a portion of ice cream or custard.

Low-fat dairy products still have all the goodness in them. They just have less fat and fewer calories.

Drinks

Drink 6–8 glasses of liquid every day to keep you hydrated and help digestion. These could include water, tea, coffee, fruit juice, fruit squash, milk and milky drinks, or occasional fizzy drinks.

WHERE DO OUR KEY NUTRIENTS COME FROM?

This chart presents the main nutrients and explains why we need them.

NUTRIENT	WHY DO WE NEED IT?	WHERE DO WE GET IT FROM?
Protein	Vital for repair and maintenance of all the cells in the body, for growth and for other functions such as the immune system.	Meat, poultry, fish, eggs, cheese, milk, yoghurt, beans and lentils, nuts, soya and other meat alternatives. We do not need a lot of protein and too much may even be unhealthy. About 4–6 oz (100–150g) a day is enough. Try to eat a mixture of animal and vegetable proteins.
Carbohydrates	To provide energy. Some carbohydrates are a rich source of fibre and vital vitamins and minerals.	Bread (including rolls, pitta, chapatti), potatoes, breakfast cereals, rice, pasta, noodles, plantains, sweet potatoes. Try to eat wholegrain cereals where possible – e.g. wholemeal bread and breakfast cereals (but not bran), brown rice. Sugar (table sugar, honey, syrup) is also a carbohydrate but is not necessary to our diet and should be eaten in moderation.

NUTRIENT	WHY DO WE NEED IT?	WHERE DO WE GET IT FROM?
Fats	An important source of energy, but eat in moderation, especially if you are concerned about weight gain. Fats enable us to absorb the fat-soluble vitamins (A, D and E). Omega-3 fats help prevent blood clots.	Butter, margarine, cream, cheese, meat, lard, vegetable oils, oily fish, nuts, seeds. Try to minimise the animal fats in your diet (e.g. butter, lard). Choose monounsaturated fats instead (e.g. olive oil, nuts). Omega-3 oils can reduce the risk of heart disease, so try to eat oily fish at least once a week.
Fibre	Helps avoids constipation; also protects against diseases such as cancer of the colon.	Wholegrain cereals, vegetables, beans, lentils and fruit.
Vitamins Vitamin A	For normal cell division, healthy eyesight and mucous membranes, and the immune system.	Oily fish, butter, cheese, carrots, apricots, green leafy vegetables, mangoes, red peppers.
B vitamins	All are needed to release the energy from foods and have other key roles too.	
Thiamin (B1)	Important role in carbohydrate metabolism.	Bread and cereal products, potatoes, pork, liver, nuts and pulses.

NUTRIENT	WHY DO WE NEED IT?	WHERE DO WE GET IT FROM?
Riboflavin (B2)	To release and support the role of other B vitamins.	Milk and milk products, eggs, meat, breakfast cereals.
Folic acid	For cell division and the formation of DNA and proteins in the body; may help to reduce the risk of heart disease.	Leafy vegetables, liver, wholegrain cereals, nuts and pulses. Try to eat more foods with this vital vitamin.
Vitamin B6	For protein metabolism.	White meat, fish, eggs, soya beans, oats and nuts.
Vitamin B12	For folate metabolism and maintenance of nerve cells.	Meat and fish in the diet. Also made by bacteria in the gut.
Vitamin C	A powerful antioxidant; also needed for healthy gums, teeth, bones and skin, wound-healing. Helps iron absorption.	Fruit and vegetables, especially citrus fruits and juices, tomatoes, potatoes, green vegetables, kiwi fruit, blackcurrants.
Vitamin D	For healthy bones and teeth: calcium cannot be absorbed without it.	Sunshine; oily fish (tuna, salmon, sardines, mackerel), fortified margarines.
Vitamin E	An antioxidant which may protect against various diseases linked to ageing.	Vegetable oils, wheatgerm, nuts, seeds, margarine.
Minerals Calcium	Keeps bones and teeth strong; also vital to blood-clotting, muscle function and nerve transmission.	Milk and dairy products, green leafy vegetables, soft bones of e.g. sardines, sesame seeds.

NUTRIENT	WHY DO WE NEED IT?	WHERE DO WE GET IT FROM?
Sodium	Maintains fluid balance within the body; important for muscle function.	Salt. We need just over 6g a day, but our average consumption is 9g.
Potassium	Keeps the heartbeat regular; maintains normal blood pressure; with sodium maintains the fluid and electrolyte balance in cells.	Bananas, avocados, fresh and dried fruit, seeds and nuts, potatoes and pulses.
Zinc	Keeps the immune system healthy; involved in the metabolism of proteins, carbohydrates and fats; may be vital to normal healing; also an antioxidant.	Seafood, red meat, milk, wholemeal bread, lentils, eggs, rice, peanuts and sunflower seeds.
Iron	Essential component of blood and vital for energy.	Offal, meat including chicken, egg yolk, dark green leafy vegetables.
Selenium	An antioxidant.	Brazil nuts, fish, offal, avocados, lentils.
Fluid	Vital for digestion, regulation of body temperature, elimination of waste products, lubrication of joints and eyes.	Water, fruit juice, milk, tea and coffee (in moderation). Try to drink more: it is almost impossible to drink too much.

SPECIFIC NUTRIENTS FOR THE OVER-50s

Some other specific nutrients are vital if we want to age well. Keeping our heart and arteries healthy has to top this list, for obvious reasons. All kinds of nutrients are needed to keep the cardiovascular system in good order (see below), but omega-3 oils deserve a special mention. These oils are now known to act on the blood platelets, making blood clots less likely.

New international research suggests they can help lower your blood pressure, too, even if you do not suffer from hypertension. With blood pressure, every millimetre counts, according to researchers. If you can reduce blood pressure by a few millimetres through eating less salt; losing a few pounds; avoiding heavy drinking; eating more vegetables, whole grains and fruit; and getting more omega-3 fatty acids, you will have made a big difference. Studies have shown that a blood pressure decrease of just 2mmHg is enough to reduce a population's average death rate from stroke by an estimated 6 per cent, and from coronary heart disease by 4 per cent.

Omega-3 oils are found mainly in oily fish such as sardines, pilchards, salmon, herring, kippers, mackerel, fresh tuna, trout and anchovies, so try to eat these at least once a week, or preferably twice. If you do not eat fish at all, add walnuts, flaxseed oil and/or rapeseed oil to your diet, as these contain some omega-3. Alternatively, take fish oil supplements to do the same job.

This book makes frequent reference to bone health (see pages 40–41, 43–4 and 145–6). It is well known that calcium is essential to keep bones healthy but current scientific opinion is that most of us are consuming enough of it. What many of us lack is the vitamin D which enables our bodies to use the calcium in food.

Our main source of vitamin D is in fact not diet at all, but sunlight acting on the skin. It is vital for all of us to get (careful) exposure to the sun in the summer months. Those who cannot get out, or who keep their skin covered, should consider a vitamin D supplement, especially in the winter (though note that vitamin D is poisonous if taken to excess). Some margarines are fortified with vitamin D. There is some evidence that high levels of protein may be bad for bone health, but no scientific consensus exists on this.

As for calcium itself, we need enough of it to protect bones but there is no evidence that a high intake helps. Calcium is found in milk (semi-skimmed has more than whole milk) and other dairy products, the soft bones in canned fish, bread, pulses, leafy green vegetables, dried fruit, nuts and seeds. A pint of milk a day will supply all the calcium we need: 700mg.

Although vitamin D is currently the 'nutrient of concern' to scientists, other research is throwing a spotlight on zinc. Zinc is involved in the metabolism of proteins, carbohydrates and fats, and having too little affects tissues that need constant renewal and repair, such as the skin, the lining of the gut and the immune system. There is evidence that older people with poor wound-healing, and particularly leg ulcers, are not getting sufficient zinc. Lack of zinc is also a factor in dementia. This vital mineral is found in meat and meat products, seafood, milk and dairy products, wholemeal bread, lentils, eggs, nuts, sweetcorn and rice.

SHOULD YOU TAKE VITAMIN SUPPLEMENTS?

Given the complexity of nutritional needs, it is tempting to add vitamin and mineral supplements as an insurance policy. These may help – or not. We simply do not have the scientific evidence yet to confirm or refute the claims made for dietary supplements. The fact that a deficiency of something is harmful does not mean that an excess of it does you good.

The current scientific consensus is that it is better to get vitamins and minerals from food. Supplements should never be a substitute for a healthy diet but may be helpful for certain people at certain times: for example, those who cannot eat properly for whatever reason, people who omit whole food groups (such as fruit and vegetables or fish) and vitamin D supplements for people who cannot get into the sun. In fact, the Canadian government has recommended that people over 65 should take a daily vitamin D supplement during the winter months, raising the prospect that the UK may one day follow the same policy.

Some scientists recommend aspirin. There is some evidence that this humble drug can help to prevent coronary thrombosis, cancer of the colon and possibly cataract too, though further studies need to be done. The precise dose has not been established: a 75-gram tablet once a day is reasonable and even one a week may be enough to gain some benefit.

Not everyone can tolerate aspirin, so it is important to check with your doctor, especially if you have gastric problems, before starting to take it each day.

A NEW LOOK AT FIBRE

Dietary fibre is an essential part of our diet that provides the bulk that helps food through the gut. Without it we do not just get constipation and haemorrhoids, we are also at risk of varicose veins, diverticular disease and possibly colon cancer. But older people should never add raw bran or bran-rich cereals or products to their diets. They contain phytates, which can bind with minerals such as calcium, zinc, iron and copper and reduce their availability in the body. Also, raw bran can simply clog up the gut, making constipation more likely. Dietary fibre is best obtained from wholemeal bread and breakfast cereals, fruit, vegetables and brown rice.

Soluble fibre is a different type of fibre. It plays a key role in how we process glucose and reduces blood cholesterol. It is found in fruit, vegetables, oats and pulses.

ALCOHOL: GOOD FRIEND, BAD ENEMY

There are many advantages to being middle-aged or older, and one of them is that alcohol is positively good for most of us. Once men have reached 40 and women are past the menopause, alcohol starts to protect the cardiovascular system because it thins the blood. The health benefits come from drinking small amounts regularly.

Modest amounts of alcohol also help to prevent gallstones, prostate problems and cognitive impairment. All types of alcohol offer these benefits: there is no truth in the notion that red wine is especially beneficial. Nor is it true that alcohol and antibiotics do not mix; only one (rarely used) antibiotic, metronidazole, should not be mixed with alcohol.

We do need to add a few 'buts', of course. If you are teetotal there is no evidence to suggest that you would benefit from starting to drink. If you do drink, alcohol should be taken in moderation, preferably with a meal. People taking prescription medicines or even some over-the-counter drugs should always check whether they are affected by alcohol. Obviously, even moderate levels of alcohol impair the ability to drive safely and can increase the risk of falls.

Moderation means a maximum of 3–4 units a day for men and 2–3 units for women (one unit is half a pint of average-strength beer, one small glass of wine in the pub, or a standard pub measure of spirits or fortified wines such as sherry: home measures are often more generous than pub measures, of course). So we can continue to enjoy drinking alcohol, but not to excess.

FLUIDS: THE FORGOTTEN FACTOR

Water is the part of our daily diet that we all tend to forget about, but insufficient fluid can cause serious problems, leading to constipation and even mental confusion. Many older people are actually slightly dehydrated. One difficulty is that the sensation of thirst declines as we age, and thirst can be mistaken for hunger, so we eat when we should drink.

We need to drink at least one and half litres of fluid a day (about six mugfuls), but we need more if we are not eating properly: for example, during illness. It is almost impossible to drink too much. Fruit juices, squash, milk, tea (in moderation) and herbal teas are all useful alternatives to water.

It is important to remember that alcohol and caffeine are diuretics: this means that an excess of them will increase the amount of water that we excrete in our urine. However, you still take in more liquid than you lose from a cup of tea, coffee or a cola-type soft drink. Try to drink a variety of drinks to keep your water intake up and remember that nothing is as good as water itself.

A QUESTION OF WEIGHT

An astonishing two out of three people over 65 living at home are overweight. Obesity makes the many disorders mentioned on pages 63–4 more likely, but it also has another damaging effect in later life: it often restricts activity. This in turn means loss of all the benefits of exercise, resulting in declining strength and cardiovascular health. Obesity also erodes the quality of life because it often leads to 'mechanical' disorders such as lower back pain, breathlessness and sleep apnoea.

It is essential to avoid weight gain – and it may be a good idea to lose weight – but as we age weight control needs to be tackled carefully. There is a big risk that restricting calorie intake drastically could affect nutritional health in other ways. The basic rules are:

- eat three sensible meals a day
- drink more water, and
- take some exercise.

It is possible to control weight by exercise alone and still enjoy puddings. If you need to lose weight, avoid crash diets. Instead, make sure you are eating a good variety of foods, but reduce the portion size, eat more slowly and up the exercise a little. Give this regime two or three weeks and you should start seeing positive results. If it does not work for you, get professional advice.

Being *underweight* in later life is not a good idea, however. Not only is there a risk of missing some nutrients but underweight people have a higher risk of osteoporosis.

HOMOCYSTEINE: THE NEW CHOLESTEROL?

Scientists are throwing a welcome spotlight on homocysteine, an amino acid found in blood which is coming to be regarded in the same way as cholesterol: too much of it may be a bad thing. It has been reported that dangerously high levels of homocysteine can increase our risk of heart disease by 50 per cent, while high homocysteine levels can amplify the risk of developing Alzheimer's disease by 150 per cent. Some 40 per cent of deaths caused by stroke have been associated with high homocysteine levels. However, direct causal links to these diseases have yet to be established, other than where there is a rare genetically induced risk.

Homocysteine levels tend to rise as we get older but are normally kept under control in the body. The control mechanisms may have a genetic basis, but they are also influenced by three vitamins: vitamins B12, B6 and folate. A deficiency of any of these three vitamins can lead to increased levels of homocysteine.

Therefore, it makes sense to keep up our intake of B vitamins to protect our hearts – and maybe our minds too. Vitamin B12 comes from meat, eggs, fish, offal and milk; folate from liver, orange juice, dark green vegetables, nuts and wholemeal bread; and vitamin B6 from potatoes, beef, fish, poultry and breakfast cereals, particularly the wholegrain variety. It is not advisable to take high daily doses of folic acid as a supplement, however, except under medical advice, as it may mask a deficiency of vitamin B12.

Meanwhile, in a recent development the UK's Food Standards Agency has been given the go-ahead to prepare plans to add folic acid to some food, such as breakfast cereals and spreads, as already happens in the USA. The primary aim is to reduce the numbers of babies born with neural tube defects, but the secondary aim is to reduce the number of people consuming too little folate, from 13.3 million to 5.6 million, without increasing the number of people with intakes above the upper limit for folic acid. You will need to read the labels to check which foods include folate.

ENJOY!

We hope you have found this dietary advice interesting and helpful. Clearly, science points the way to healthier choices in our diet. But we humans are complex beings and there are centenarians alive and kicking who have never followed any of the rules.

There is one overriding rule about food: enjoy it. There is little point in changing from your usual diet if doing so will undermine your appetite for food – and even life itself. Do what you can to eat wisely, and get on with your life.

MEAL IDEAS

Try to eat regularly, at least three times a day. If there are times when you do not feel like cooking, choose instead from the wide variety of canned, chilled and frozen 'ready meals' now available. Stews and soups are particularly easy to make and you need only one pot to cook them in.

Many people with low incomes are convinced that they cannot afford to have a healthy diet – but eating healthily doesn't have to be expensive. Try to buy fruit and vegetables that are in season, when they should be cheaper. If you buy fresh fruit and vegetables that are sold loose, you will not need to buy large quantities of one item.

All food, whether hot or cold, provides warmth and energy. A snack can be just as nourishing as a more traditional meal. Here are some suggestions:

BREAKFAST FOODS
- toasted currant teacake and a milky drink
- fruit – fresh, canned, dried (or fruit juices)
- crumpets, muffins or toast with butter and jam or cheese
- peanut butter or banana sandwich and fruit juice
- hard-boiled egg and toast
- cheese and tomato on toast
- yoghurt (try it with muesli, honey and fresh fruit)
- pancakes with grilled bacon and tomato
- wholegrain breakfast cereal, for example, a wheat- or bran-based kind, or porridge.

MAIN MEALS
- spaghetti bolognese with green salad
- corned beef hash with green vegetables
- roast chicken with potatoes and vegetables
- cauliflower or macaroni cheese with bread and salad
- boiled bacon with parsley sauce and broad beans
- steamed or baked fish with potatoes and vegetables
- spinach and potato curry with chapattis or boiled rice
- omelette with potato and vegetables
- meat or bean casserole with swede and cabbage
- liver and onions with mashed potatoes and carrots
- shepherd's pie or fish pie with peas and green beans
- vegetable stir-fry with noodles.

QUICK AND EASY MEALS

- sandwiches – try tuna, cheese, corned beef, peanut butter, hummus, ham or egg and salad
- toast – with pilchards, well-cooked scrambled egg, baked beans, creamed mushrooms or canned spaghetti
- jacket potato with cottage cheese or grated cheese and baked beans
- soup containing meat or pulses (such as lentil, beef broth or pea and ham) with grated cheese and wholemeal bread
- sausages, baked beans and instant mashed potato
- kippers or smoked haddock with bread and butter
- pitta bread with hummus, pepper, celery and carrot
- pasta and bean salad (try using kidney beans, chickpeas, butter beans, tomato and lemon juice).

PUDDINGS AND DESSERTS

- fresh, canned or stewed fruit
- fruit crumble or pie with custard or cream
- ice cream
- jelly or mousse
- yoghurt
- sponge and custard
- rice pudding.

SNACKS

If you feel like a snack during the day, try fruit, a small handful of unsalted nuts or seeds, breakfast cereal with milk, or cheese and crackers. You could also try toast with low-fat butter or margarine, jam, cheese or peanut butter or have a milky drink. Or you could have a fruit smoothy – try blending a banana and other soft fruit such as peaches or strawberries with some orange juice or milk.

STORE CUPBOARD ITEMS

It is useful to have a store of basic foods, in case there is ever a time when you cannot get to the shops. Here are some suggestions:

- milk – long-life, dried or evaporated milk; canned milky puddings
- meat and fish – canned corned beef, ham, sardines, salmon, pilchards, mackerel and tuna
- fruit, vegetables and fruit juice – a variety of canned fruit and vegetables (including tomatoes and baked beans), dried fruits, lentils and other dried beans and peas, long-life fruit juice, instant mashed potato and frozen vegetables
- cereals – breakfast cereals, wholegrain crackers, plain biscuits, pasta and rice
- drinks – tea, coffee, cocoa, malted milk
- canned and dried soups; yeast extract (for example, Bovril, Marmite or Vegemite); stock cubes.

If you have a freezer, you could use it to store a small supply of foods you enjoy: for example, frozen mince and chicken pieces, frozen vegetables, a selection of 'ready meals', frozen seasonal fruit and ice cream. It is a good idea, when cooking a stew or homemade soup, to freeze individual portions. You can then defrost the meal for eating when you feel like it.

Buy only food that you will use. Store cupboard foods don't keep forever, so use them occasionally and replace them with new ones. Don't let things go out of date.

OVERCOMING OBSTACLES TO EATING WELL

It is not always easy to maintain a good diet in later life, for all kinds of reasons. There are often simple solutions to the difficulties, however.

Even if we are well motivated to eat sensibly, getting older can put obstacles in our way. Shopping and cooking may become more difficult, our taste buds are becoming less sensitive – so food may become less interesting – and dental problems may compound the disincentive to eat well.

Simple strategies can help. For example, we do not need to be able to cook well to eat well. A sandwich can become a nutrition-packed meal with the right fillings. Things to grill on toast include tomatoes (a rich source of lycopene), or sardines (a great source of omega-3 oils) and calcium, if you eat the soft bones. Convenience meals that can be heated in the oven or microwave cooker can be nutritious, if expensive. However, watch out for meals that are high in fats, salt or sugar: there are often healthier options.

Social factors are critical, as research has shown. Cooking for one is a challenge at any age and people who have a partner or friends to eat with have a better diet than those who live and eat alone. So try to build enjoyment into food by eating with your family and friends, at home or in a café or lunch club.

LOOKING AFTER YOUR TEETH

Research has shown that older people who do not have their own teeth are more likely to be malnourished than those who do. So it pays to hang on to our teeth for as long as we can. The advice on avoiding too much exposure to sugar, which rots teeth, brushing regularly, and visiting the dentist for regular check-ups applies at all ages. Gum disease is often the cause of lost teeth: we should brush our gums gently and see the dentist if our gums bleed.

If you suffer from dry mouth, speak to your dentist or doctor about it. Some medicines can cause dry mouth as a side-effect, and some medical conditions may affect the salivary glands, so that they do not produce enough saliva. Drinking plenty of fluids can help, as can sucking a sweet or chewing gum – but make sure these do not contain sugar. You may be prescribed artificial saliva in spray form to help moisten the mouth, or your doctor may be able to switch your medication.

If you wear dentures, make sure they fit properly. Our jaws change as we get older, so dentures need to be changed from time to time. ■

5

MINDING THE BRAIN

MINDING THE BRAIN

People worry more about mental decline in later life than they do about physical ill-health. But research shows that although some memory and other lapses are normal, significant mental decline is not inevitable and there are things we can do to support brain function and mental health. The brain is actually much more dynamic than was once thought.

AGE, MEMORY AND UNDERSTANDING

If you cannot find your house keys, have forgotten the name of your new neighbour and catch yourself looking for the milk in the microwave, do not worry – this is quite normal. (We should start worrying only when these lapses become severe.) Studies have shown that everyday 'cognitive deficits', such as forgetting things, start to creep in from about the age of 45. Younger people forget things, too, of course – and we do not put their lapses down to age.

Cognition comprises all the mental processes that enable us to perceive, remember, think and solve problems. Working memory – the span of immediate memory that, for example, enables us to remember an address while we write it down – declines with age. Working memory is a key component of cognition as it affects reasoning, calculation, speaking, listening, reading and writing. Long-term 'episodic' memory – our memory for personal events – also declines. However, semantic memory – the basic understanding we have of our world – holds up very well. The very oldest are as good as the youngest in remembering that fires are hot, birds sing and the world is a sphere. None the less, as we get older we take longer to retrieve things from memory, partly because there is interference from so much irrelevant material in our brains. We also know that older people process information more slowly.

These observations are of course based on averages. Studies

have shown that there is immense variation in cognitive ageing; in some people, cognitive abilities hold up extremely well, while in others they decline quite sharply. In many cases, decline in cognitive ability is linked to physical ill-health. It is, for example, common during what is known as 'terminal drop', the last two to three years of very late life among people with multiple diseases and difficulties. Other factors may affect cognitive ability too, such as deafness and possibly sight defects.

If this sounds dismal, it is not. Mental deficits may be irritating but they are rarely precursors of something more sinister. We do not lose our capacity to perform everyday cognitive tasks, or even to learn complex new skills or acquire new knowledge (unless a disease intervenes). We just take longer to get there. And there are strategies to support cognitive performance, and indeed to support brain health.

HOW TO RETAIN BRAIN POWER

How do we set about keeping our brains as young as possible? Science does not have all the answers yet, but there are things we can do which definitely help and there are 'insurance policies' that may be worth taking out.

TAKING A LOOK AT THE BRAIN

Studying the ageing brain was a real challenge until the invention of imaging techniques, such as magnetic resonance imaging (MRI), in the late 1970s. These techniques allow neuroscientists to 'peer inside' the living brain as it undertakes various mental processes. There is still much to unravel about the complexities of this mysterious organ, but what we now know should give us all a rosier view of just how durable and adaptable our brains are.

Our brains comprise billions of cells – neurons, or nerve cells – each in constant communication with other neurons. In the cortex alone, where memory is stored, there are thought to be 100 billion cells, with 13 trillion connections between them. In the tiny gaps between neurons – the synapses – all the biochemical activity takes place to transmit messages from one neuron to another, enabling us to think, act and feel. Several chemical messengers called neurotrans-mitters are activated in the synapses to pass the messages along. So far, scientists have discovered more than 40 neurotransmitters and it is thought that others will be found. They include, for example, dopamine and serotonin, both key players in our moods.

However, things can go wrong in the interactions between the neurotransmitters. Even subtle changes in brain chemistry can have profound effects. For example, lack of dopamine causes the symp-toms seen in Parkinson's disease, which affects movement of all kinds, from walking to smiling, while low levels of serotonin are associated with depression.

All the neurotransmitters depend on oxygen and glucose; although the brain accounts for only 2 per cent of body mass, it uses 25 per cent of blood oxygen and a massive 70 per cent of available glucose. Simply to survive, it uses a tenth of a calorie a minute. In contrast, when you are walking to the shops, your body burns about four calo-ries a minute. But if you are really concentrating, such as when doing a crossword puzzle, the brain uses 1.5 calories a minute.

There are plenty of outdated notions about the brain that we need to discard. First, we need to stop believing that we are born with practically all the brain cells we will ever have, that no more new ones develop beyond our teenage years, and that the brain can-not repair itself. It is now known that neurogenesis, or the creation of new neurons, continues in the adult brain – every day the rat's brain generates as many as 9,000 new neurons – and it has been shown that many of these new neurons survive and integrate them-selves into the working brain. In effect, the brain contains its very own class of stem cells. The new neurons survive through support from neighbouring glial cells (the second type of brain cell), nutrients from the blood and, most importantly, through connections with other neurons. Without these connections, they wither and die.

Findings to date suggest that neurogenesis mainly takes place in the hippocampus, which lies deep in the brain and is involved in learning and memory. Two other areas where it is most evident are the caudate nucleus, involved in motor control, cognition, the emotions and learning, and the olfactory bulb, through which we detect odours. Now, the hunt is on to find ways of turning on neurogenesis, with the aim of establishing new ways of treating Parkinson's disease.

Researchers at Princeton University in the US have also found a link between poor levels of neurogenesis and depression, which can reduce the size of the hippocampus. What is more, they say, chronic stress, even without full-blown depression, can damage the hippocampus, working against the production of new cells. (Other work using antidepressant therapy found that it stimulates neurogenesis in adult animals.) The Princeton researchers have also found that in Cushing's disease – a tumour of the pituitary gland, which sits at the base of the brain and helps in regulating hormones – a depressed hippocampus can lead to loss of memory.

Interestingly, there is evidence from animal studies of strong links between learning and new neuron survival. After teaching rodents a variety of tasks that engaged a number of different brain areas, researchers found that, generally, the more the animal learned, the more neurons survived in the hippocampus. Animal experiments have also shown that exercise is as good for your brain as it is for your heart. Mice that used a running wheel had about twice as many new hippocampal neurons as mice that did not exercise. The current thinking is that learning may still be necessary to preserve them.

So far, therefore, researchers have identified areas of the brain where neurogenesis is evident, and discovered processes that may promote or inhibit it. We also have a glimpse of how new neurons may assimilate into the working brain. But many important issues remain to be explored.

For example, do the new cells replace old neurons, or do they set up completely new circuits? Are the findings in animals relevant in humans? As yet, it has not been possible to prove this conclusively – our current imaging capacity is not yet capable of getting down to this cellular level. But Swedish researchers carrying out post-mortems on people who died of cancer have found evidence of new cells in their brains.

There is also work going on that is designed to find lifestyle answers as well as medical ones to some of the conundrums of the brain. The Disconnected Mind is a study being run by the University of Edinburgh in partnership with Research into Ageing (the biomedical research programme within Help the Aged), which follows up the people who took part as children in the Scottish Mental Survey. This was carried out among all 11-year-olds in Scotland in 1947, to explore their mental abilities and background. It was never repeated. Now, 60 years later, some 1,000 of the original participants have agreed to take part in a further eight-year trial (lasting until 2015) to probe into what makes people mentally healthy or unhealthy. They will retake the same mental aptitude tests they did in 1947, and undergo MRI scans and DNA and other biochemical tests.

So we can expect a sequence of valuable findings over the coming years that will shed new light on how the brain ages. Professor Ian Deary, leader of the Edinburgh team, is using new methods to test the hypothesis that mental decline is caused by a mix of damage to the protective 'white matter' that encases the brain's nerve cells, and a breakdown in the connective circuits, literally causing the brain to become disconnected.

The trial will also examine the relationship between blood circulation and dementia, and look for signs of a relationship between diabetes and dementia. Other issues that are likely to come into the picture are the effect on the brain of lack of exercise, and an explanation of why wounds heal more slowly with age.

Already, work carried out in the build-up to the main study has shown that smoking has an adverse effect on information-processing, verbal learning and memory. Also, people who took vitamin supplements did better in cognitive tests; however, their 1947 results showed that the same people were typically brighter than most. So it looks more as if bright people take vitamins, rather than that vitamins make people bright. We will know more as the study progresses.

Research elsewhere has highlighted the importance of folic acid supplements in slowing down age-related cognitive decline and in its positive effects on ageing and some dementias. The recommended daily dosage for maintaining good health is 400 micrograms, but in a three-year study on slowing cognitive decline, participants were taking 800 micrograms a day.

Note, too, that the government will shortly be allowing foods such as bread to be fortified with folic acid (see page 80), so if you would like to begin taking a folic acid supplement it is best to check with your doctor about what dosage would be appropriate for you.

PHYSICAL EXERCISE: THE BRAIN PRESERVER

What we do know is that moderate physical exercise has a direct effect on some neurotransmitters. Exercise of at least 30 minutes stimulates the production of serotonin, low levels of which are associated with depression. We can all feel the effects of serotonin after exercise because a 'feel-good' sensation sweeps over us, making us feel more energetic and cheerful. Exercise also releases endorphins – natural painkillers that give some people a 'high' when they exercise. Animal experiments have shown that exercise also increases levels of dopamine and, as already mentioned, that it plays a role in neurogenesis.

Exercise has other brain benefits too, including the stimulation of the proliferation of blood vessels in the brain and an increase in synaptic connections between brain cells.

Clinical trials have shown that exercise programmes can help people with depression, enabling them to reduce and even to come off antidepressant drugs. People who take up exercise report feeling more alert and certain types of exercise – yoga and *t'ai chi*, for example – help to reduce anxiety. Regular exercise lowers blood pressure and keeps the arteries healthy, thus protecting against vascular dementia.

Other studies have shown that 'super-fit' older people have very little cognitive decline. It is certainly a good insurance policy – if nothing else – to take regular exercise for the sake of our brains as well as our hearts and muscles. And, of course, a good diet plays a major role, too.

LEARNING TO HELP THE BRAIN

Older people who have regular mental stimulus appear to maintain their cognitive abilities better. There is some evidence that people with higher levels of education have a lower risk of Alzheimer's disease. Old rats given new toys to play with positively fizz with new neuronal connections and increased blood flow to the brain, and what is true of old rats may also be true of humans. But we do not know exactly what we should be doing, for how long and with whom (social activity may be better than doing the crossword on our own, for example), to keep our brains in good shape.

All the same, it is a good insurance policy to keep up all levels of mental stimulus – it will not harm and it might help our brains. A lifetime committed to new experiences, learning and playing probably enhances our mood and that is vitally important in later life. Studies have shown that the people who live the longest are generally those who are most content and most involved in the life of their communities.

As for coping with memory deficits, memory can be trained to some extent and we can learn strategies to support our forgetful minds, whether it is making lists or using imagery to help. It also helps to enhance other skills, such as concentration. We cannot remember what we did not see or hear properly and we will get on more quickly with any task if we focus on it. As we get older, our minds are ever-bigger warehouses of thoughts, feelings, memories, worries and other distractions that can get in the way of action. Our older brains, however, are also an immense storehouse of experience that we can draw on – and share.

For example, the range of opportunities for volunteer work is huge nowadays – anything from helping young children improve their reading skills, through to utilising professional expertise in, say, engineering, teaching or healthcare in projects carried out abroad (where expenses and a local wage would probably be paid) or on shorter projects such as an archaeological dig, for which you pay. For more information, see the www.do-it.org.uk website.

There is also the University of the Third Age (U3A), which has over 630 groups around the country and about 185,000 members. They are all run independently by volunteer tutors who are themselves members. Again, the interests covered range from archaeology to walking, and there is a national summer school. The idea is to learn for the sheer pleasure of learning – there are no assessments or qualifications to be gained.

The Open University's Open Learn website, at www.open.ac.uk/openlearn, is free of charge and offers a huge range of subjects, including short courses on work-related subjects as well as leisure interests such as writing (fiction, family history, and so on), photography and personal finance. Other courses constitute complete units taken from the formal university programme, including modern languages. It is an interactive site, so you can link up with others using the material if you wish, wherever they are in the world.

If you are none too sure of your computer prowess, ask for the free Help the Aged advice leaflet entitled *Computers and the Internet* (also available via www.helptheaged.org.uk), or try www.silversurfers.net, a site specifically for anyone over 50 who wants to find out about the internet and how to use it.

The latter is also a mine of information on all sorts of topics, from health to travel. It is run in conjunction with Digital Unite, which has its own site at www.digitalunite.net, offering tuition in how to use a computer, aiming particularly at 'hard-to-reach' people, such as those living in residential care. The idea is for everyone to feel comfortable with technology. And take heart – in 2002, the oldest person learning to use a computer was a lady of 108 living in Yorkshire.

WHY MENTAL HEALTH MATTERS

Mental illness can affect us at any age but the most common disorders in older age, such as depression, are treatable. Diagnosis is the first step – never put mental problems down to 'old age' and ignore them.

It goes without saying that mental health *does* matter most of all to us as individuals. No one wants to contemplate a future of depression or anxiety or, worse, a condition such as Alzheimer's disease. Mental frailty of one sort or another will, however, also affect other aspects of our health. People who are forgetful, confused or suffering from mental illness are least likely to be getting a good diet, which adds to the risk of physical illness and may make the mental problems worse. Indeed, self-neglect is often a sign of a mental health problem of some kind. We do not know what effect poor mental health has on normal exercise patterns, but it is likely that exercise needs are also neglected, with all the health risks that brings.

Families and friends are another important factor in this equation because it is often they who have to cope with the effects of mental health problems. The stresses involved in caring for someone who is very confused or has dementia are well known and it is often mental frailty that leads to people entering residential care.

For all these reasons it is vital to maintain mental well-being. It is also important to recognise that only a minority of older people suffer from serious mental decline or mental illness. It is simply not true that we all get dementia if we live long enough. So what can we expect 'at our age', what can go wrong and how can we preserve our mental health?

WHAT CAN GO WRONG?

DEPRESSION

Depression affects about one person in eight among those over 65. Older people are, in fact, more likely to have mild depression than any other age group, though this is not because older age is inherently depressing. It is because depression is often a side-effect of physical illness and other knocks, such as bereavement or divorce. Whatever lies behind it, depression can seriously affect quality of life, not only for patients but also for their partners and families.

At times we can all feel a bit low or even downright miserable. These feelings are a natural reaction to life's worries and sadness, but we gradually resolve them and recover. Clinical depression is very different.

People with depression may experience a range of symptoms, including lack of energy and motivation, loss of concentration and poor memory, feelings of hopelessness, irritability, agitation, sleeping problems and loss of appetite. Depression is often accompanied by persistent tiredness and sometimes by unexplained pains, particularly headaches and abdominal pains. For these reasons, many people assume they have a physical illness and it is often this that makes them consult a doctor. Sometimes depression affects behaviour – sufferers may become aggressive, start shoplifting or misbehave in a sexual way.

There are different kinds of depression. Some people become depressed in the winter months when daylight hours are short: this is known as 'seasonal affective disorder' or SAD. Bipolar disorder, as manic depression is now known, is rare, characterised by swings of mood from very low to elated. But most people are simply described as having a 'depressive illness'.

Unlike an ordinary episode of 'feeling low', clinical depression, if untreated, may last for months or even years or, in severe cases, may drive people to suicide.

Depression may be triggered by bereavement, distressing events or anxieties, or may simply come out of the blue. As many as 60 per cent of people who have a stroke develop depression afterwards. There may also be links between other illnesses and depression; heart or lung disease and dementia may trigger it, and it is a non-motor symptom of Parkinson's disease.

Depression is not a personal failing: it is an illness. The good news is that it can be successfully treated, so do not hesitate to go to your doctor. One problem with depression in later life is that it may go unrecognised and untreated, leaving people to suffer needlessly. It is vital to realise that with help you can recover. Regardless of whether depression occurs out of the blue, or following another illness such as stroke, it usually responds well to treatment.

AVOIDING DEPRESSION

Currently we do not have a full understanding of what causes depression, but some things may reduce the risk. Exercise has already been mentioned as a key factor, and diet is also important. People who are short of B vitamins are at risk of depression, while it is now thought that omega-3 oils, found in fish, also play a significant role. People who have seasonal affective disorder can be helped by exposure to special 'light boxes' (for other reasons, we all benefit from higher light levels at home, and from exposure to the sun). For people who have had one episode of depression, the best way to avoid another is to stay on antidepressant medication.

Social factors are all-important in depression, however. Friendships, family relationships, purposeful activity – these are our best defence. Anything that enhances mood and self-esteem is also worth doing, whether that is luxuriating at the hairdresser's, having a face-lift, taking up painting, buying a kitten or trawling the internet for new friends. In retirement we need to plan for what will take the place of paid work and the stimulus, purpose and companionship that it offered.

'Age is opportunity', as Longfellow wrote, and we need to work at opportunities for fun, friendship and support in later life.

DEMENTIA

There are several types of dementia: Alzheimer's disease is the most common. Dementia can affect people of any age, but is most often found in older people. One in 14 people over 65 has a form of dementia, and this rises to one in six of those over 80.

Dementia is a devastating and progressive condition, which means that symptoms become more severe over time. It starts with a decline in mental ability, which affects memory, reasoning and communication skills, eventually accompanied by a gradual loss of the skills needed to carry out daily activities. The way each person experiences dementia, and their rate of decline, will depend on the type of dementia they have, their physical make-up and emotional resilience, and the support that is available to them.

Researchers are still working to find out more about the different types of dementia. The three most common forms are Alzheimer's disease, which accounts for 62 per cent of dementias, vascular dementia, and a combination of vascular dementia and Alzheimer's.

It is thought that many factors including age, genetic background, medical history and lifestyle can combine to lead to the onset of Alzheimer's disease. Vascular dementia is caused by problems with the supply of oxygen to the brain following a stroke or small vessel disease.

While there is no fail-safe way to prevent dementia, it does appear that a healthy lifestyle and diet could reduce the risk. Meanwhile, research is continuing into developing drugs, vaccines and treatments. Aricept, Exelon and Reminyl are existing drugs that can temporarily alleviate some of the symptoms of Alzheimer's in the early to middle stages. They act in the brain to maintain supplies of an important chemical called acetylcholine. Also a newer drug, Ebixa, has been developed, which can be helpful for people in the middle to later stages of Alzheimer's.

There is evidence for the possible protective effects of statins, which lower cholesterol (hence helping to keep the circulation healthy) and may also directly affect the brain. Other studies are looking at non-steroidal anti-inflammatory drugs (NSAIDs) such as aspirin; the B vitamin folic acid; and Ginkgo biloba, an extract from leaves of the maidenhair tree.

A number of vitamins or medicines have anti-oxidant properties and it is suggested that these might help to prevent brain damage caused by free radicals, which are produced by normal brain activity. However, the jury is still out on this, especially as some, such as vitamin E, could increase the risk of stroke and hence of vascular dementia. For similar reasons, experts are also still divided about whether hormone replacement therapy could increase or decrease dementia risk.

There is much to gain from further scientific research. Both the Help the Aged biomedical research programme Research into Ageing and the Alzheimer's Society are continuing to fund important research in this area.

Help the Aged produces a free advice leaflet on mental health (also available via www.helptheaged.org.uk). ■

6
WHAT CAN WE EXPECT AT OUR AGE?

WHAT CAN WE EXPECT
AT OUR AGE?

Ageing brings a whole series of changes and challenges, but one of the latter is knowing what is normal at our age and what should send us scurrying to the doctor. Here is what we can expect.

STILL FIRING ON ALL CYLINDERS

Ageing can be described as a progressive loss of efficiency and adaptability. We can still fire on all cylinders, but as faults begin to occur in our cells and cellular mechanisms most of our bodily functions become less efficient and less able to deal with the stresses that we would once have taken in our stride.

For example, wound-healing is slower, and because our immune systems are operating less effectively we take longer to bounce back from infections such as flu or bronchitis. Old lungs are less elastic and the usable volume of air is reduced. Muscle strength declines and the heart pumps less effectively. That is why a fit 70-year-old marathon runner will complete the course in four hours while a fit 20-year-old can do it in two.

People in their 80s and even their 90s do indeed participate in and complete marathons (you do not actually have to run the 26 miles, 385 yards: walking is quite acceptable), proving that age itself is no barrier to health and fitness. Illness is more likely but few conditions are inevitable. A healthy older person should expect only the following.

SKIN CHANGES
The skin becomes less elastic and thinner as we age, but wrinkles have more to do with exposure to the sun than to age as such.

HAIR CHANGES

Hair loses its colour and thins in both women and men. The age at which this happens is genetically determined. But as our skin gets gradually paler with age, if we are colouring our hair we will need to adjust the shade to a slightly lighter tone to stay as natural-looking as possible.

TEETH WEARING OUT

Teeth are vulnerable after a lifetime of wear, but with care they can last the distance. Make sure you regularly eat some crunchy raw fruit and vegetables, to keep jaws and teeth in good working order. We are not great at looking after our teeth, though – for some years now, in the UK, only just over half of us (57.7 per cent) have been receiving dental treatment. And more than half of over-65s in Scotland have lost all their teeth.

NHS dental provision has become a scarce commodity over the last few years, which has not encouraged people to go for regular check-ups – and has even led to some people removing their own bad teeth with pliers. If you are having trouble finding a nearby dentist willing to do NHS work, contact your local primary care trust (PCT). You will find the details by accessing www.nhs.uk.

EYE CHANGES

The lens in the eye becomes less elastic, making it harder to focus on near objects (presbyopia) and the eyes take longer to adjust to changes in light levels.

We need higher light levels as we age – aim to get 400 watts into every room, especially in areas such as stairs, or anywhere else where the floor level changes, where there is a risk of trips. And if we live long enough we are likely to get cataract, but this is because exposure to the sun degrades the proteins in the lens. In the UK an estimated 42 per cent of people aged over 75 develop cataracts.

Having a cataract is a bit like viewing the world through a dirty car windscreen, which causes light beams to be scattered and creates a blurred image. Cataracts usually form slowly, with a gradual deterioration of vision. When these problems make normal daily activities difficult, it is time to get the cataract operated on. Cataract can be cured by a simple operation. Make sure you have eye tests every couple of years – they are free from the age of 60.

Age-related macular degeneration (AMD) is another eye condition that affects people over the age of 50. It is not painful, although it is the most common reason for people over 65 being registered blind or partially sighted in the UK. It affects the central part of the retina, a light-sensitive layer inside the eye that converts into signals the light that comes in through the pupil. These signals are then carried by the optic nerve to the brain to enable us to see.

The macula enables us to see colour, and what is straight in front of us, as well as the fine detail, such as printed text and people's faces. If the macula degenerates, we lose the central part of our vision. This makes it difficult for people with the condition to read or watch television and recognise faces. However, their side (or peripheral) vision remains intact and, with practice, can be enough for people to maintain an independent life.

AMD tends to develop in two ways. 'Dry' macular degeneration is caused by a build-up of waste products in a layer of cells below the retina. This type of macular degeneration, into which 85 per cent of cases fall, usually progresses slowly over several years. Both eyes can be affected, although symptoms may develop in one eye long before the other. It is not known why the pigmented cells lose the ability to process waste and there is no known treatment for 'dry' macular degeneration.

About 15 per cent of people who develop AMD have 'wet' macular degeneration, which often develops quickly and causes severe damage to the eyes' central vision. The disease can affect both eyes but not necessarily at the same time. Once a person has developed 'wet' macular degeneration in one eye, their chances of developing it in the other eye increase year on year. The likelihood of this happening varies, depending on the specific kind of damage that is developing in the affected eye. There are currently two treatments that may help delay the decline in central vision and they both involve lasers.

Researchers agree that smoking definitely increases the chances of developing AMD. There is also a genetic link to the condition, so it makes sense to have your eye health checked regularly if you have a blood relative who has developed AMD.

HEARING IMPAIRMENT

Hearing loss is common, particularly at high frequencies – about 50 per cent of people over 65 are deaf or hard of hearing. The scientific jury is still out on whether this is the result of ageing processes, our genes or a lifetime's exposure to noise.

Hearing loss becomes much more common as we get older, with more than half of people over 60 experiencing problems, and 30 per cent having to use hearing aids. The progressive loss of hearing that occurs with age is known as presbycusis, and is thought to be caused by changes in the cochlea.

The cochlea, found in the inner ear, is shaped like a snail's shell and contains tiny hair cells which move in response to the vibrations passed from the ossicles (small bones in the middle ear). The movement of these hair cells generates a signal that is transmitted to the brain. We are born with about 16,000 hair cells in the inner ear, but as we get older we gradually lose them and we don't have the ability to regenerate them. Presbycusis is a progressive condition, but people do not usually notice any effects until well after 50.

Hearing loss frequently has an adverse effect on older people's quality of life. It creates feelings of frustration, social isolation and loneliness, which can all lead to lower self-esteem, withdrawal and depression.

At present there is no cure. Treatments rely on hearing aids and

LOOKING AFTER YOUR HEARING

1 Never poke anything into your ears, not even cotton buds. This can push wax down on to the eardrum, where it can cause damage.
2 Use a flannel and plain water to clean the outer surface only.
3 See the doctor if you have an infection or blockage in the ear.
4 Be careful of the damaging effects of loud noise; one result could be tinnitus, an irritating persistent sound in one or both ears that tends to be worse at night.
5 Wear ear protectors if using noisy equipment.
6 Do not turn up the volume of personal music systems or other sound-producing appliances too far.

If you suspect that you or your partner are suffering hearing loss, try the RNID's five-minute hearing check (see chapter 10 for the telephone number), or go to your GP.

The earlier hearing loss is diagnosed, the easier it is to prevent it from getting worse.

Unfortunately, many people wait up to 15 years between the onset of hearing loss and seeking advice about it. This makes it more difficult to adjust to a hearing aid's amplification as they have got used to a 'quieter' world.

cochlear implants, which are electronic devices inserted into the inner ear that send sound-generated electrical pulses directly to the brain.

Modern digital hearing aids are very effective and discreet, and in principle they are now available on the NHS, but waiting times to have one fitted are still lengthy. Some 30,000 people in England have been waiting for up to two years for a first hearing test, while 500,000 people with an analogue hearing aid are waiting for a digital replacement. Meanwhile, PCTs have been urged by the Department of Health to speed up the queues, using private sector facilities if necessary. Audiology practitioners, as found in high street shops, may be brought in to help reduce the delays. It is hoped that if these sorts of measures come into force, the backlog will disperse.

FOOT PROBLEMS

These tend to increase later in life. Many of us tend to neglect our feet until they start giving us trouble. About 75–80 per cent of the adult population has a foot problem.

Feet are certainly put through their paces. The Society of Chiropodists and Podiatrists reckons that the average person walks the equivalent of five times around the earth in a lifetime and, in simple walking, each step can exert up to twice your body weight in ground reaction force through your lower limb, meaning that a 10-stone person will have between 15 and 20 stones of impact going through the heel on each heel-strike. That is pretty punishing treatment by any standards.

So what can we do to prevent problems? For a start, we can wear properly fitting shoes, something that is easier said than done – not least because the general fitting of shoes and boots for adults has not changed over the last 50 years, even though our body shapes have. Women in particular tend to be taller and heavier now than they were half a century ago. The width of the shoe should correspond with the widest part of the foot while standing. We should allow 1cm on the length of the longest toe to give our toes wiggle room, and because we all have one foot slightly longer than the other (usually the left foot) it is important to go for the longer measurement.

Unfortunately, at least a third of women have feet wider than the standard width for their size, so what tends to happen is that they buy a larger size to get the breadth. Thankfully, some manufacturers have recognised this problem and are making shoes to fit today's feet. Emotion (www.emotionshoes.co.uk) is one such, specialising in making stylish footwear for women specifically for the wider foot and calf, at high street prices. It is best to avoid completely flat shoes, as they do not support the foot; go for a 1–1$\frac{1}{2}$ inch heel. A good pair of trainers will also incorporate this lift, with the heel moulded inside. Moderately high wedge-heeled shoes are fine, too, as they support the general shape of the foot.

Ill-fitting or inappropriate footwear can lead to problems. Wearing the wrong sort of shoes to work, for instance, such as high heels when you do a lot of standing, or not wearing safety footwear with a steel toecap if your occupation requires it, can result in burning sensations, lack of feeling, tingling or cramping in the feet and toes, caused by poor circulation, or swollen feet, ankles or legs, as well as bunions, calluses and corns. In fact, the ill-effects of standing for long periods can reach beyond the feet, ankles and legs to the knees and hips, and the back and neck too.

Foot problems can also result from injury – objects falling on to your feet, an accident while wearing slippers that are loose or worn out, falling on slippery floors – or be a complication of a disease such as diabetes, where poor blood circulation to the feet can affect nerve response there and lead to loss of sensation. Foot problems also worsen some conditions, increasing the pain of rheumatoid arthritis, for example.

Looking after your feet means washing them every day with soap and water, rinsing them and drying them thoroughly, especially between the toes. Cut your toenails straight across, to avoid painful ingrow-

EXERCISE YOUR FEET

Exercise can really help to keep feet healthy – it tones up muscles, helps to strengthen your arches and stimulates blood circulation. Try doing the following exercises regularly.

1 Rising on tiptoes

Stand with feet parallel and, holding on to a steady piece of furniture for support, rise slowly up and down on your tiptoes. This exercises the leg muscles and helps strengthen the foot muscles.

2 Point your toes

Sitting down, extend and stretch the foot in as straight a line with the leg as possible.

3 Rotate your feet

Still sitting, extend feet one at a time and rotate slowly at the ankle, as if you are trying to draw the largest circle possible with your big toe. Do this first in one direction, then the other.

4 Wiggle your toes

Remain sitting with feet resting on the floor. Move your toes up and down.

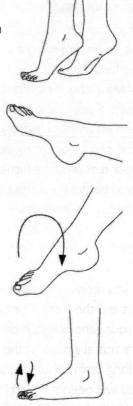

ing toenails (it may be easier to do this in the bath, once the nails have softened a little in the warm water), and do not cut them too short. Massage moisturising cream into the feet after washing them, but not between the toes; any moistness here can lead to the fungal infection athlete's foot. For the same reason, do not wear the same shoes for two days running, to allow the sweat to dry out properly, and change your socks or tights every day.

Exercises to keep your feet and ankles supple and strong include circling each foot in turn ten times in each direction, keeping the leg as still as possible. Pick up a pencil with the toes of one foot, and place it down next to the other foot; repeat with the second foot. See the text box opposite for more foot exercises.

Walking about barefoot at home is good, as long as the flooring is safe. If you are standing all day, try to move about, shift your stance from one leg to the other, or flex the feet up and down to keep the circulation going. At home, lie down for 15 minutes a day with your feet and legs higher than your head and heart.

If you have painful feet, see a chiropodist or podiatrist for advice. You may have to go privately, though, as podiatry services have been greatly reduced in recent years by many PCTs, owing to financial constraints.

Under the NHS, each case is assessed individually and whether or not you receive free treatment depends on how serious your condition is and the risk factor. Low-risk problems which are unlikely to affect your general heath or interfere with your mobility may mean you are not eligible. On the other hand, people with diabetes and other long-term conditions are treated as priority cases.

You will need a referral from your GP, practice nurse or health visitor. Go to www.nhs.uk to find out whether your local PCT funds chiropody treatment. If not, your GP can still refer you to a private clinic, where you will have to pay. If you are contacting a chiropodist yourself, check that they are fully qualified and registered with the Health Professionals Council (HPC) and a member of a recognised organisation, such as the Society of Chiropodists and Podiatrists. (In case you are wondering, the essential difference between the two terms is that strictly speaking 'chiropody' refers to both feet and hands, while 'podiatry' is the internationally recognised name for a foot specialist and refers just to feet. Podiatry also reflects a new type of training which extends the chiropodist's skills and expertise, including carrying out day surgery in some instances.)

Incidentally, for non-invasive bunion treatment, you can ask your GP to refer you to the Marigold Clinic at the Royal Homeopathic Hospital in London, which can also put you in touch with podiatrists trained in the same special technique and practising outside London. The technique is not based on homeopathy but rather on herbal treatment, involving the application of a paste made from the *Tagetes* marigold (the French marigold), for its anti-inflammatory properties. In a 1996 trial of 60 bunion patients, the paste was more effective than placebo. (Note that some PCTs have stopped NHS referrals for homoeopathic treatments at the hospital, on the grounds of lack of effectiveness, so you may have to emphasise that this is herbal treatment. Private patients currently pay £100 for a first consultation, £75 a time thereafter.)

MENOPAUSE DISORDERS

Somewhere between the ages of 47 and 52, women reach the menopause, when periods stop and the protective amount of oestrogen produced by the ovaries reduces over time. This means that cardiovascular function, collagen (the scaffolding that supports skin and bone) and bone itself become more vulnerable.

About 70 per cent of women will experience troubling symptoms owing to hormonal imbalances. Classically, these include hot flushes, vaginal dryness, night sweats and mood swings. These generally disappear within a couple of years, but in some women the discomforts can go on for very much longer.

In fact, the ovaries do go on producing some oestrogen for about five years after the menopause, while some is produced from the adrenal glands, and some is manufactured in body fat.

Despite the scary headlines it has generated, hormone replacement therapy (HRT) is not entirely out of the picture. The trick is to use it as a short-term aid; the risks associated with oestrogen are cumulative.

It helps to put the risks in perspective. For every 10,000 women who are not on HRT, you can expect that every year 30 will develop heart disease, 30 will contract breast cancer, and 21 will have a stroke. If they are on combined HRT (this form is not given to women who have had a hysterectomy), then there will be seven more cases of heart disease, eight more breast cancers, and eight more strokes.

If a close family relative (mother or sister) has suffered a heart attack or breast cancer, you may not wish to opt for HRT. On the other hand, being obese increases the risk of breast cancer more than taking HRT.

For women under 50 who have an early menopause it is a rather different scenario. First of all, the risk of heart disease and cancer is lower in younger women; secondly, in these cases the HRT is only restoring their hormone levels to the natural levels they could have expected up to the age of 50.

It is best to discuss your own situation with your doctor, so that you can make an informed decision about whether or not to take HRT. And your doctor can advise on how to gradually wean yourself off it when the time comes, perhaps by taking it every other day or by cutting patches in half.

Given all the scares over HRT – usage has dropped by half – it is not surprising that many women are looking for alternative treatments to help. The best way to start is to look closely at what you are eating. Make sure you are eating oily fish a couple of times a week for their omega-3 fatty acids, and some nuts and seeds every day. Eat phytoestrogens – contained in soya, chickpeas and lentils – as they help to balance your hormones and can help lower your cholesterol levels. Keep up your intake of fruit and vegetables for their antioxidant properties, and the fibre they contain. Eat unrefined foods such as brown rice and wholegrain bread. And do not give up on the exercise, which helps in preventing osteoporosis by maintaining bone density.

Some women turn to herbal treatments to alleviate their symptoms. But a word of caution: if you are already on medication for something else, ask your doctor for advice before going ahead. The most commonly used remedies to help relieve sweats and flushes include black cohosh (however, note that recent findings suggest that taking it long-term may have toxic effects on the liver), or vitamin E and evening primrose oil. *Agnus castus* (the chasteberry) or vitamin B6 supplements can help with mood swings.

HORMONAL CHANGES IN MEN
Sex hormone activity declines with age in men, too, and though this may be gradual, some men may be aware of an 'andropause', or male menopause, taking place quite quickly.

Symptoms include fatigue, reduced sexual and physical drive, erection problems, irritability and depression, memory loss, joint stiffness and excess sweating, especially at night. It is not so much a question of falling testosterone levels, more a matter of how sensitive or resistant the body has become to testosterone.

What happens is that proteins that bind testosterone start to accumulate, and this reduces the amount available to the body. And low testosterone activity can play a part in high blood pressure and cholesterol levels, which can lead to heart and circulatory problems, especially if the man is overweight or has diabetes.

Experts in men's health believe that the symptoms and their degree of severity are a better indicator of reduced testosterone activity than the blood test men are likely to be offered by their GP, since this measures total testosterone rather than under-activity. Dr Malcolm Carruthers, for example, suggests a three-month trial of testosterone replacement therapy in the first instance, to see if the symptoms disappear.

Testosterone replacement should not be regarded as a cosmetic anti-ageing technique, though, and for this reason should only be taken under medical supervision. There is growing evidence that it protects against metabolic syndrome (a cluster of the most danger-ous heart risk factors), Alzheimer's disease, cardiovascular disease and depression, and we can expect preventive strategies using testos-terone replacement to emerge in due course.

Recent findings related to erectile dysfunction (which now includes the older term 'impotence') suggest that physical reasons rather than emotional ones are the cause in 75 per cent of cases. Increasingly, too, erectile dysfunction is being recognised as an early-warning marker of potential health issues such as metabolic syndrome, car-diovascular disease, diabetes and depression.

It is important to get checked out by your doctor rather than resorting to Viagra on your own, so that these potential problems can be picked up if necessary. Having said that, the use of Viagra, Cialis or Levitra, the three drugs for erectile dysfuncton, combined with testosterone treatment restores full erections in 70 per cent of cases, according to Dr Carruthers.

A useful self-help guide to men's health can be found at www.male-health.co.uk, a website run by the Men's Health Forum and partially funded by the NHS.

PROSTATE DISORDERS

By the age of 60 most men will have prostate problems. Benign prostate hyperplasia (BPH) is the non-cancerous growth of the prostate gland, possibly caused by reduced testosterone activity, which results in difficulty and discomfort in passing urine. Do not put up with it, because it can be successfully treated. If you are being tested for this, make sure your GP does both a PSA (prostate-specific anti-gen) blood test and a rectal examination to screen for prostate cancer.

You can also ask to be screened for prostate cancer under the Prostate Cancer Risk Management Programme, which is available to men who do not have any symptoms but still want a blood test. This is not a national screening programme as such, though, since major trials being carried out have yet to show how effective large-scale PSA screening would be in terms of reduced illness and death.

Meanwhile, the programme allows men to discuss having a PSA test with their GP and, after weighing up the pros and cons, they can have one free on the NHS if they wish. Doctors advise annual PSA screening for men aged 40 with a family history of prostate cancer, and for others from age 50, ideally built into other men's health checks.

It is worth noting that urinary tract infections in men can cause PSA levels to shoot up.

◆ ◆ ◆

And that, largely, is it. Relatively few conditions are directly attributable to age. In the next section we list some of the symptoms you should definitely not put down to your age and ignore.

WHEN YOU MUST SEE THE DOCTOR

What follows is not intended to cover everything that can go wrong but it sets out some of the symptoms that older people all too often put up with in the mistaken belief that we can expect no better 'at our age'.

In most cases, your doctor will be able to help – very few conditions are untreatable. Under the National Service Framework for Older People, which defines standards of care for major medical issues, there is also a new emphasis on helping older people to stay well or to maintain quality of life while living with a chronic condition. So do not be fobbed off by doctors who think that older people are inevitably unwell or less deserving of healthcare resources – we are entitled to good healthcare at any age.

Some symptoms are so obviously signs of illness that we will not describe them here – things like bleeding from any orifice (including the gums), sudden loss of weight, diarrhoea, lumps and bumps. However, there are potentially serious conditions like high blood pressure (hypertension) that may have no obvious symptoms. It is for this reason that we urge everyone reading this book to take advantage of the MoT-type services that doctors offer.

In Scotland, the official policy is to offer everyone a health check at age 50, and every five years after that. Elsewhere, 'Well woman/man' clinics at the local surgery will identify conditions such as hypertension and diabetes before they cause real damage. GPs are expected to review the medication of everyone who is on repeat prescriptions. For anyone aged 75-plus who is on long-term medication, this should be an annual review; for people on four or more medications, it should be six-monthly. And if you have not needed to see a doctor by the time you are 75, make sure you go along then for a health check.

We should also see the optometrist (optician) at least every two years and the dentist every six months; as well as checking eyes and teeth, these professionals can identify conditions you would not associate with their field. For example, an eye test can show up the presence of a brain tumour. And do not forget to make use of the national screening programmes that are now available to you (see pages 24–7).

Pain is a symptom that something is going wrong and should always be taken seriously. Pain in your chest, abdomen or head should always be investigated. Joint pain may be caused by arthritis, and although this is common in later life, it is a still a disease and can be treated. Exercise or physiotherapy should be part of the treatment regime for people with osteoarthritis. Some pain, however, is the result of disuse or misuse rather than disease – back pain being the main one. Back pain may indicate a need for exercise that enhances spinal strength and flexibility, attention to posture or even a new bed.

Breathlessness may indicate that we are out of condition or it may indicate a chest problem, anaemia or a heart problem. Always check it out.

Falls on a regular basis are a sign of something going haywire. The major accompanying risk is that you could well sustain a fracture as a result. Your balance or muscle strength may be the cause, and exercise can put these right, or your sight may be impaired so you cannot see obstacles too clearly. If you do not know why you fell, it may indicate a heart problem. It is vital to get a proper assessment if you have more than one fall, and that may need to include seeing a cardiologist.

As discussed on pages 143–6, osteoporosis may be diagnosed following falls leading to fracture of the wrist, hip or spine, particularly in post-menopausal women. Now, under the National Service Framework for Older People, your GP and PCT should be putting greater emphasis on helping people to avoid falls, and integrating this with the local osteoporosis services. They should also be improving these services, by providing DEXA scanning and, if necessary, organising a risk assessment at your home, to advise on safety measures that would help.

Unfortunately, at the time of going to press only about half the health authorities had reached this standard of service.

Some of the practical things you can do at home to prevent falls include mopping up spills straight away, making sure there is no clutter around the place and organising cupboards and the like so that you minimise the need to climb, stretch or bend to find things. Various types of aids can also help, if necessary. You could have a fall alarm system installed, or consider wearing a hip protector beneath your clothes – they can reduce the risk of hip fracture by some 50 per cent. Your GP can advise.

Confusion and extreme forgetfulness are not normal, however old we are. They can be symptoms of many things. Confusional states can be triggered by nutritional deficits, dehydration, infections (urinary tract infections often go undiagnosed in older people), thyroid problems or other physical illness, as well as mental illness. Anyone suffering from confusion needs a thorough medical assessment to find the cause and provide relevant treatment. The confusion often recedes once the underlying problem is fixed.

Vitamin B12 deficiency is thought to affect about 10–20 per cent of the population, but is probably more common in later life than the statistics suggest. B12 helps to provide the body with healthy nerve cells and red blood cells. It is also involved with helping to form the DNA needed for new cells. But although it is an important nutrient, we cannot manufacture it ourselves; it has to be taken in from animal-derived food, notably meat (particularly liver), shellfish and milk products. It is also found in fortified breakfast cereals – and in Marmite. This means that strict vegetarians who do not touch meat, fish or dairy products are at particular risk unless they take the fortified cereals, where the B12 derives from plants, and possibly a B12 supplement on top.

We need a daily intake of only 2.4 micrograms, so inadequate intake is not usually the reason for deficiency. More often it results from disturbances in the way we absorb B12. It comes attached to proteins in our food, and its absorption requires the stomach to first secrete a protein called intrinsic factor, so that the B12 can then be released by stomach acid and absorbed. As we get older we produce less intrinsic factor, and so become more vulnerable to chronic B12 deficiency.

Another cause may be medications that reduce levels of stomach acid. Examples include anti-ulcer drugs such as ranitidine or omeprazole, and metformin, used to control Type 2 diabetes. Deficiency can also develop following stomach surgery or other types of digestive disorder. Check out with your doctor whether a daily supplement is needed.

One difficulty with diagnosis is that the symptoms tend to develop slowly, and are easy to mistake for all sorts of other conditions. Early on, cognitive function is likely to be marginally reduced. Eventually, anaemia develops. Other symptoms may include tiredness, sleep problems, weakness, constipation, loss of appetite and weight loss. There can also be numbness and tingling in the hands and feet, a sore mouth or tongue, difficulty in maintaining balance, poor memory, depression, confusion and dementia. It is now thought that folate and vitamin B12 work together to protect cognitive function, although this has yet to be proved conclusively, but it does seem to be vital to keep them in balance.

Researchers at Tufts University in the USA found that people of 60 and older with normal B12 levels and high levels of folate in the blood had satisfactory scores in cognitive function tests assessing response speed, sustained attention, visual spatial skills, associative learning, and memory. But people with low B12 levels and high folate levels performed poorly, and were found to be five times more likely to have anaemia and cognitive impairment than those with normal levels of B12 and folate.

Loss of sight indicates an urgent trip to the doctor – or nearest casualty department if it is sudden. The sooner you get treatment for some eye conditions, like glaucoma, the more likely it is that your sight can be saved.

Another eye condition to be aware of is age-related macular degeneration (see page 107), a major cause of deteriorating eyesight in which the ability to see properly when looking straight ahead is lost, and you are dependent on peripheral eyesight. Age is the main factor for this condition, with genes accounting for about 50 per cent of cases, smoking for about 29 per cent, and the remainder thought to be caused by lifestyle factors such as a high-fat diet and excess alcohol intake.

Incontinence is commonplace and distressing – about 6 million people in the UK are affected – but it is not inevitable. Women are particularly at risk, though for many the cause is slack pelvic floor muscles which can be tightened up again by suitable exercise. It is best to see a professional first for advice on exercise, as it is very difficult to learn exercises correctly from a leaflet.

Do not be embarrassed to discuss the problem with your doctor and make sure he/she takes a proper medical history, so that the cause of your incontinence can be identified. Ask to be referred to a specialist incontinence nurse or a physiotherapist specialising in women's health; men tend to be referred to a urologist instead, even when the nurse could advise. Alternatively, you can refer yourself directly to the specialist nurse. Some run clinics in GP surgeries, or they may work in community hospitals or community centres. Unfortunately, they are distributed unevenly around the country, so contact your PCT or the Continence Foundation for the nearest one to you.

Apart from pelvic floor exercises, treatment may involve advice on your fluid intake and other lifestyle factors, bladder retraining or slow-release medications for an over-active bladder. Incidentally, many specialist incontinence nurses are entitled to prescribe the medications.

Help the Aged produces a free advice leaflet, *Bladder and Bowel Weakness*, on managing incontinence (also available via www.helptheaged.org.uk).

See also information on pages 124–5.

Constipation tends to occur in later life because the gut is more sluggish. However, it is often the result of faulty diet, insufficient water or lack of exercise.

Do not attempt to cure it with added bran in your diet (see page 76) and try to avoid laxatives on a regular basis. See your doctor about a strategy that works and keeps you off pills.

BLADDER AND BOWEL WEAKNESS

Incontinence becomes more common as we age and seriously affects the quality of many older people's lives.

Getting rid of your body's waste products is a complex process. When our control mechanisms don't work properly, incontinence – the accidental or involuntary leakage or urine or faeces – is the result. This can have an impact on confidence and well-being as well as on personal hygiene and health.

What causes incontinence?

Ageing cannot cause incontinence. Although bowel and bladder weakness becomes more common as we get older, incontinence is not an inevitable part of ageing, but as it is not a distinct disease it is often difficult to determine the cause.

Types of urinary incontinence

There are four kinds:

- **stress incontinence** – leaking urine when you cough, sneeze or exercise. It is caused by weakness in the muscles that control the opening of the bladder as well as the pelvic floor muscles. This type of incontinence is most usual in women because of the impact of pregnancy, but men may develop it after a prostate operation.
- **urge incontinence** – having a sudden urgent need to pass urine, but not being able to reach the toilet in time. An overactive or 'unstable' bladder can be the cause.
- **overflow incontinence** happens when the bladder does not empty completely. Urine can build up and end up 'overflowing'.

■ **functional incontinence** – in which practical issues such as having difficulty walking or not being able to undo clothing quickly enough can lead to incontinence.

Faecal incontinence

Losing control of one's bowels is distressing and embarrassing. Sometimes the cause is malfunction of the nerves at the base of the spine that control the lower bowel. Damage to the sphincter muscles in the anus, or to the nerves controlling these muscles, or constipation can also cause bowel leakage. Pelvic floor weakness is another leading cause, and this can also contribute to urinary incontinence.

What to do about incontinence

See your doctor. Otherwise, try to drink normally (6–8 cups of liquid a day), but cut down on caffeine (tea and coffee); avoid constipation by eating plenty of fibre, and try to keep as active and mobile as possible.

Sleep problems – these are a very common reason why people over 65 go to their doctor. Chronic lack of sleep can really undermine our quality of life and it lowers the immune system, too. A common cause of poor sleep (for partners as well as patients!) is sleep apnoea, when we briefly stop breathing then start again with a thunderous snore. Ask to be referred to a sleep specialist if you find your difficulties are becoming severe.

Sleeping problems can be the result of medical conditions that affect the bladder, such as diabetes or prostate problems. Stress, anxiety or pain (which often seems worse at night) are other common causes. Or it could be that our circadian rhythm – the biological body clock that regulates our personal 24-hour activity/rest cycle – is out of synch. The way we respond to a changed circadian pattern can vary; we might find ourselves sleeping in shorter bouts, or waking up extra early.

Another type of response could be nocturnal polyuria, when we scarcely wee during the day but need to get up at least twice at night. Here, what is thought to happen is that the body's daily secretion of arginine vasopressin is disturbed. This is a hormone that increases the resorption of water from the kidney, so reducing the volume of concentrated urine.

Now, work at the University of Glasgow is shedding new light on what is happening when our circadian rhythm is disturbed. Our body clock is controlled in the brain by the hypothalamus and age-related changes produce deficits in some of its neurochemical transmitters, changing how some behavioural signals respond to light wavelengths, for example. In turn, these deficits have an impact on the way that associated chemicals act – one consequence is that the immune function and other processes are not running in synch. The researchers are looking to see whether they can increase the activity of the chemicals that are not in deficit, to compensate for those that are.

Professor Stephany Biello has some practical advice for people who cannot sleep. These tips should help to restore your normal circadian pattern:

- get outside during daylight hours
- do not read or watch TV in bed – the bedroom is for sleep and sex
- if you cannot sleep, get up, move to another room and do something else
- whatever you do, get up at the right time in the morning. This improves the likelihood of sleeping properly the next night.

Stress can afflict us at any age and we are not immune once we are retired. Stress in older people may in fact be clinical depression, a highly treatable illness (see also page 99). It is not good practice to deal with anxiety states by signing up for a lifetime of tranquillisers. It is worth talking to your doctor about alternatives.■

7

CONDITIONS WE CAN (LARGELY) AVOID OR IMPROVE

CONDITONS WE CAN (LARGELY) AVOID OR IMPROVE

Science has helped us to understand how we can prevent many illnesses that become more common as we get older. Research shows that our genes can make certain conditions more likely – for example, people from South Asian ethnic groups or with a family history of heart disease are at greater risk of suffering cardiovascular disease. Our environment and luck play a part, too. But we inherit more than genes. Unhealthy behaviour can also be passed down the generations. If you are at risk of any of the illnesses described below, consider whether you could make a change to give added life to your years.

To help in this, try out NHS Choices at www.nhs.uk, a resource specifically designed to inspire people to achieve a healthier life by putting them in charge of decisions about their own health, lifestyle and treatment options. Its Live Well section provides information to help the well to stay well and to advise on living with specific long-term conditions, and the content can be accessed by gender and age, to reflect individual needs.

Another new development is that you could find that you have been called in for assessment by your doctor. The National Institute for Health and Clinical Excellence (NICE) is suggesting that family doctors comb surgery records for patients with a high risk of developing heart disease or stroke within ten years, with a view to giving them advice on how this could be prevented.

In any case, everyone over 40 should have their blood pressure taken at least every five years – and make a note of the reading so that they can regularly check that it remains within an appropriate range (either with a home monitor or at the pharmacy). Keeping an eye on your blood pressure is important, because the higher your blood pressure the greater the risk of developing narrowed arteries, which could lead to heart problems, kidney disease or strokes.

But you will not necessarily be aware of any symptoms even if your blood pressure is consistently high.

Blood pressure levels are in fact only one of several factors doctors take into account when deciding whether someone needs treatment for high blood pressure (hypertension). Just as important are lifestyle habits. So make sure you are not overweight, do not smoke, do not drink more than the recommended daily intake of alcohol, watch your (saturated) fat intake and also your salt consumption. We need only six grams of salt a day – a teaspoonful – but on average we consume nine grams, mostly through processed foods and salty snacks. (The government is trying to reduce this to six grams, while some experts advise three.) Take regular exercise and try to deal with any stress you may be experiencing.

Blood pressure is expressed as two readings. The first number is the systolic pressure, which indicates the maximum pressure in the system; the second is the diastolic, or the lowest pressure in the system. If you have no known coronary disease and your reading is less than 140/90, you will not need treatment. If it is between 140/90 and 159/99, you will be advised to alter your lifestyle. At 160/100 and beyond, you will be put on medication.

For patients with coronary heart disease, the levels are different. If your blood pressure is 140/85 or over, you will be prescribed medication. Diabetics with coronary heart disease will be given medication at readings of 130/80 or more.

But do not worry if your blood pressure seems a little higher when a doctor takes it compared with other times. Doctors are well aware of this 'white-coat' phenomenon and do make allowance for it. In any case, they will take several readings on different occasions before making a diagnosis of hypertension.

There are two other types of blood tests which it pays to have regularly checked – your cholesterol and homocysteine levels. Both substances are produced naturally in the body, where they have important functions, but in both cases too much can be a bad thing.

It is a matter of keeping the levels under control.

In the case of cholesterol, about 80 per cent is manufactured by the liver, with 20 per cent coming from your diet. Low-density lipoproteins (LDLs), mostly from saturated fats, carry the cholesterol around in the blood, and may deposit it in the body, and it is this build-up that can lead to problems. High-density lipoproteins (HDLs), which are derived from poly- and monounsaturated fats, carry the cholesterol back to the liver, so removing it from the blood and protecting your heart. LDLs and HDLs are commonly referred to as 'bad' and 'good' cholesterol respectively, but it is more correct to think of them as neutral, since both are needed by the body. Good health depends on the correct balance between them — which means you need to keep your LDLs low and your HDLs high.

Blood cholesterol levels are measured in millimols of cholesterol per litre of blood (mmol/l). It is difficult to suggest standardised appropriate levels, as these vary according to age, gender and general health. But anyone over 40, or who has a family history of raised cholesterol, should know their level. If you are generally healthy but have a raised level, start by reducing your intake of saturated fats (animal fats, full-fat dairy products, palm oil taken in through cakes and biscuits) and increase your intake of monounsaturated fats (olive oil, nuts, avocados), and polyunsaturated fats (sunflower oil, oily fish). Avoid like the plague hydrogenated and partially hydrogenated fat. Depending on your personal history, your doctor may also prescribe cholesterol-lowering medication, such as statins.

Much the same applies to elevated homocysteine levels. This is an amino acid produced in the body by the chemical conversion of methionine, a compound we take in through eating methionine-rich foods, such as fish. The methionine is taken into the bloodstream and into cells, where it is changed into homocysteine, which is basically toxic if not processed properly; blood levels that remain high can cause serious problems. The correct processing produces further chemical changes which are entirely beneficial.

The desirable changes produce a chemical called S-adenosyl methionine (SAMe), which is a useful natural antidepressant, fights against arthritis and helps to lower homocysteine levels. As levels of SAMe increase, this causes glutathione, another vital chemical, to be produced from homocysteine. Glutathione is the body's best anti-ageing agent and also acts as a detoxifier. A low glutathione level has been linked to an increased risk of death from all common causes. So once again the message is to keep the homocysteine level down and the glutathione level up.

There is mounting evidence that to do otherwise is to court disaster.

Homocysteine levels are measured in micromols per litre of blood. A 'safe zone' is generally considered to be below 9 μmol/l although, as with cholesterol, there is no healthy level for homocysteine as such. Anything above 14, and you are considered to be at major risk of suffering a heart attack or stroke, and you have an increased risk of Alzheimer's.

According to the Alzheimer's Society UK, at least one in two people die prematurely from potentially preventable diseases, and more than one in two people have elevated homocysteine levels. World Health Organization estimates suggest that dangerously high homocysteine levels increase the risk of a heart attack by 50 per cent, while the American Heart Association has found that 40 per cent of deaths from stroke are linked to high homocysteine levels.

The AHA has also established that a homocysteine level above 14 μmol/l amplifies your risk of developing Alzheimer's disease by 150 per cent. Other conditions in which elevated homocysteine levels are implicated include concentration and under-achievement (impaired cognitive performance), osteoporosis, diabetes and pregnancy complications. The upside is that patients with levels below 9 who have undergone coronary angioplasty treatment suffer from significantly fewer new arterial blockages and cardiovascular disease later in life.

Homocysteine levels tend to rise as we get older but are normally kept under control in the body, as already indicated. The control mechanisms may have a genetic basis, but they are also influenced by three vitamins – vitamins B12, B6 and folate (folic acid). A deficiency of any of these three vitamins can lead to increased levels of homocysteine.

So it makes sense to keep up our intake of B vitamins to protect our hearts and our minds, too. Vitamin B12 comes from meat, eggs, fish, offal and milk; folate from liver, orange juice, dark green vegetables, nuts and wholemeal bread, and vitamin B6 from potatoes, beef, fish, poultry and breakfast cereals, particularly the wholegrain variety.

Dietary supplements are another route to increasing your intake. According to Dr Marilyn Grenville, research suggests that the best amounts to take to reduce homocysteine levels are 500 micrograms of vitamin B12, 25–50 milligrams of vitamin B6, and 0.5–5 milligrams of folic acid. It is not advisable to take high daily doses of folic acid as a supplement, except under medical advice, as it may mask a deficiency of vitamin B12.

The good news is that a 3 μmol/l drop in homocysteine levels reduces the chance of heart attacks by 16 per cent, strokes by 24 per cent and deep vein thrombosis by 25 per cent. A 5 μmol/l drop reduces the risk of death from all causes by 49 per cent, death from cardiovascular disease by 50 per cent, and death from cancer by 26 per cent.

Some doctors consider that homocysteine levels are a more reliable indicator of health status than cholesterol levels and that dietary cholesterol in and of itself is not the critical link to heart disease risks that we once thought. We have not heard the end of this debate.

DIABETES: A NEW EPIDEMIC

Diabetes is increasing at an alarming rate and doctors now regard it as the one of the world's most serious diseases. It is characterised by raised levels of blood glucose because of a deficiency in the production and/or action of the hormone insulin. When insulin cannot control the processes that make glucose available to the tissues where it is needed, such as muscle, the tissues are starved of energy even though there is plenty of fuel available.

Type 1 diabetes is characterised by a lack of insulin production and accounts for about 5–15 per cent of all diabetes cases. It tends to start at a young age and is controlled by daily insulin injections throughout life.

Type 2 diabetes, also known as non-insulin-dependent diabetes, was until recently found mostly in adults, but it is now also occurring in obese children. It accounts for 85–95 per cent of all diabetes cases. With this type, insulin is being produced but the body becomes insensitive to its action, and the pancreas cannot secrete enough insulin to keep pace. Insulin resistance may also be involved in heart disease and high blood pressure. When first diagnosed, diet and exercise alone may be sufficient to control blood glucose levels in Type 2, but management of the condition tends to change over time, with the addition of oral medication. Some patients will also be prescribed insulin. Indeed, many doctors consider that early insulin therapy is important in minimising long-term complications in Type 2 diabetes. However, going on to insulin therapy may result in weight gain, and diabetics are urged not to cut back on insulin to lose weight. Instead, if you have this disorder, stay in close touch with your diabetes team, who will be able to advise you on an appropriate weight-loss programme based on exercise and diet and ensure you are on a modern form of insulin, where weight gain is far less of a problem.

Over 2 million people in the UK have diabetes, and an estimated further 750,000 have it but do not yet know it. Those at particular risk include people with a family history of diabetes, Asians and African-

Caribbeans, and people who have a large waist – over 80cm (32in) for a woman and 92cm (37in) for a man. Unfortunately, because the onset of Type 2 can be insidious, it may be several years before people are diagnosed with it, when complications have already set in. And the complications of Type 2 diabetes can be every bit as severe as those of Type 1.

Prolonged exposure to raised blood glucose levels damages tissues throughout the body by affecting the blood vessels and on average, life expectancy is reduced by more than 15 years in Type 1 diabetes, and by between five and seven years (at age 55) in Type 2. Adults with diabetes have heart disease death rates about two to four times higher than adults without diabetes, and the risk of stroke is also two to four times higher. About 30 per cent of people with Type 2 diabetes develop overt kidney disease.

Other types of complications can include peripheral vascular disease (which may lead to amputations), cataract and a blinding eye disease called diabetic retinopathy, and ulcers on the feet and legs caused by damage to the nerves. Diabetics are more susceptible to the ill effects of other risk factors such as smoking and high blood pressure. Yet in most cases diabetes can be avoided. Some people have a genetic risk of diabetes but even they can take steps to minimise the risk.

The causes of insulin resistance are not well understood but there are two major risk factors for Type 2 diabetes – obesity and inactivity. If we want to avoid diabetes we should aim to get our weight to a reasonable level and, most of all, we should take regular, moderate exercise.

Exercise acts directly on the metabolism to ensure that our body is sensitive to the actions of insulin. Exercise can even help those with a strong family history of diabetes and those who already have the condition. The type and frequency of exercise are important in this context. It must be aerobic (that which makes our heart and lungs work harder) or weight-bearing exercise, and it must be done regularly in at least half-hour blocks, though this can be split into 10- or 15-minute bursts. People who have diabetes should aim to exercise at least every three days because the effects of exercise wear off.

CARDIOVASCULAR DISEASE

You are as young as your arteries, goes the saying. And it is not only our hearts that benefit from healthy arteries.

The heart is designed to beat 31 million times a year for over 100 years and all it asks is a regular supply of oxygen and nutrients via the arteries. We have to mention smoking first. Carbon monoxide from smoking reduces the ability of the blood to carry oxygen to the heart and all other parts of the body. Nicotine stimulates the body to produce adrenaline which makes the heart beat faster and raises the blood pressure, causing the heart to work harder. People who smoke have twice the risk of a heart attack of those who do not. If you do smoke, stopping will be the best single thing you can do to help your heart – not to mention your lungs and many other organs. Moreover, the benefit to your heart starts as soon as you stop smoking.

Exercise is key to a healthy cardiovascular system. Exercise improves the 'electrical stability' of the heart, making heart attacks less likely. It strengthens the heart muscle and keeps the arteries elastic, both of which enable more oxygen to reach the brain, muscle and other tissues. Exercise lowers blood pressure and blood cholesterol levels, and increases insulin sensitivity (see pages 135–7 on diabetes). If you are at risk of any heart disorder, talk to your GP about 'exercise on prescription', usually available through your local authority (see page 38).

In terms of diet, it is crucial to eat the right fats and to lower the intake of all fats, while the anti-oxidants found in fruit and vegetables are also vital for cardiovascular health. Fats high in saturates (such as butter, cheese, the fat in meat, lard) increase the levels of LDL. It is

HEART ATTACK SYMPTOMS

Chest pain or pressure is the most common symptom of a heart attack, but **not everyone who has a heart attack experiences pain.**

In addition to chest pain, symptoms may include:
- a tightness or squeezing sensation in the chest
- arm pain (often the left arm, but it can be either)
- upper back pain
- sweating
- headache, toothache or jaw pain
- shortness of breath
- nausea, vomiting, and/or discomfort in the upper/middle abdomen
- heartburn and/or indigestion
- generally feeling ill.

However, in about 25 per cent of heart attack cases there are no symptoms. The heart attack without symptoms is particularly common among diabetics.

Note that even if there are no symptoms or the symptoms appear to be mild, such heart attacks can be every bit as serious as ones where extreme pain has been experienced.

It is essential to seek medical help immediately: early treatment could save your life, while a delay could lead to permanent damage to the heart.

this which sticks to the walls of the arteries, clogging them up (atherosclerosis). Depending on which arteries become blocked, the result may be a heart attack, angina, stroke, kidney failure or limb ischaemia (poor blood supply to the legs causing pain on walking).

Monounsaturated fats can help lower LDL levels and do not lower HDL. Olive oil, walnut oil and rapeseed oil are monounsaturated fats and some margarines and spreads are made from them. The British Heart Foundation advises combining monounsaturated fats with polyunsaturated fats, such as sunflower oil, corn oil, walnuts and soya and sunflower seeds, as this helps to stabilise the improved levels. Omega-3 fats can help prevent blood clotting, and are found in fish oil and oily fish such as pilchards, sardines, salmon, mackerel and trout. If you do not eat fish it is worth taking a fish oil supplement.

Medication may also have a place in helping to prevent cardiovascular disease. Your GP may prescribe a statin drug, for example. Statins are increasingly being used to reduce the risk of having a heart or stroke event by reducing cholesterol levels. They are also known to reduce the risk of a further attack in people who have already suffered one. There has been a welcome downward shift in the death rate from cardiovascular disease and no doubt some of this can be ascribed to people taking better care of themselves. And because treatment is also improving, it means more people today are living with heart disease.

STROKE

We should be as concerned about 'brain attacks' – for that is what strokes are – as we are about heart attacks. Stroke is the third-biggest killer in the UK, after heart disease and cancer. Strokes are disabling in many ways: they can cause physical disability, are the cause of about 20 per cent of all dementias and frequently result in depression.

Nine out of ten strokes are caused by exactly the same processes that lead to a heart attack or angina. Plaque deposits in an artery in or leading to the brain cut off the blood supply, or sometimes a clot forms somewhere else and travels to the brain, with the same effect. This type of stroke is linked with high blood pressure, smoking, high blood cholesterol, diabetes, heavy drinking, lack of exercise and being overweight.

Strokes can also be caused by a burst artery in the brain – and the commonest cause of bleeding into the brain is high blood pressure. Depending on which part of the brain is affected, the outcome may be paralysis, loss of balance, slurring or loss of speech, difficulty swallowing, loss of bladder control, memory problems, dementia and loss of vision.

One serious and under-recognised complication of stroke is depression. This affects more than half the people who have a stroke and can be a major obstacle to recovery. Depression is a perfectly normal psychological reaction to the losses caused by stroke, but it may also be that when the brain is injured the survivor may not be able to experience positive emotions.

Atrial fibrillation, or an abnormal heart rhythm, is very common in the over-60s, and increases with age. It is also a leading cause of stroke, as the irregular heartbeats lead to blood stagnation and so increase the risk of blood clots that may travel from the heart to the brain and other areas. Patients are often given anticoagulants such as warfarin to protect them from strokes, and are strongly advised not to smoke and to cut down on caffeine.

It is worth asking your doctor for a risk assessment if you have symptoms such as palpitations, fainting or chest pain, but often there are no symptoms. Atrial fibrillation can be treated with medications to slow the heart rate or to revert the heart rhythm to normal, or with cardioversion, where a tiny electric shock is administered to the heart. Certain patients may be fitted with a pacemaker to stabilise the heart beat, others with an ICD (implantable cardioverter defibrillator) if they are at risk of life-threatening abnormal rhythms.

REDUCING THE RISK OF STROKE

There is no single underlying cause of stroke. Risk factors can include existing medical conditions such as high blood pressure, high levels of cholesterol, diabetes, heart disease and thickening of the arteries (arteriosclerosis). If you have or think you may have any of these conditions see your GP and ask advice on how to minimise your risk from stroke.

Lifestyle changes that can help to reduce the risk from stroke and improve your general health include:

- giving up smoking
- drinking alcohol only in moderation
- doing regular physical exercise
- keeping your weight at a sensible level
- eating a healthy diet, low in fat, salt and sugar and high in fruit and vegetables, and
- having your blood pressure checked at least once a year.

For more information about stroke, contact the Stroke Association (see chapter 10).

RECOGNISING STROKE

The sooner someone is diagnosed and treated after experiencing a stroke, the better the outcome is likely to be. But the symptoms of stroke can be easily missed, leading to delays in seeking help.

The Face Arm Speech Test (FAST) has been developed as a stroke identification instrument, which can be used by non-medical people to assess the three neurological signs of stroke:

1 Ask the individual to SMILE.
2 Ask them to RAISE BOTH ARMS.
3 Ask them to SPEAK A SIMPLE SENTENCE (coherently), such as 'It is sunny out today'.

If the person has trouble with any of these tasks, call an ambulance.

A severe stroke may be fatal. However, many stroke patients make a reasonable recovery, especially if expert treatment is started quickly. If you suspect someone is having a stroke (the signs often include slurring of speech or sudden weakness down one side), call your doctor immediately. In recent years there has been a government-spurred drive to establish more specialist stroke units, and to develop other available stroke services.

OSTEOPOROSIS

Osteoporosis is a condition that affects the bones, causing them to become thin, fragile and liable to break. It affects about 3 million people in the UK. It is a painless condition and for most sufferers the first they know of it is when they fracture an affected bone, most commonly in the wrist, hip or spine. Women are particularly at risk but men can get the disease, too. Fortunately, osteoporosis is almost always avoidable.

Bone is a living tissue that is constantly being replenished. By the age of 35 we have reached 'peak bone mass' and after that we start to lose bone at a slow rate; women, however, lose bone faster after the menopause. If we lose too much bone it is prone to fracture in vulnerable places and fractures can even occur spontaneously, especially in the spine. Osteoporotic fractures can be catastrophic, not least because we may lose confidence in our ability to function independently.

Calcium and other minerals in our food are the raw materials used in the bone-forming process, so diet plays a big role in preventing osteoporosis. We need an adequate intake of calcium, which comes from foods including milk and dairy produce and green vegetables such as broccoli. Avoid fizzy drinks, which interfere with calcium absorption. However, scientists believe that calcium intakes are generally sufficient in the UK and what is lacking in our diet is the vitamin D that enables us to use the calcium. Vitamin D comes principally from sunshine acting on the skin, and it is advised that we get exposure to the sun on as many days as possible in the summer months. For bone health, we should go easy on caffeine, sodium and protein, all of which encourage the excretion of calcium through the urine. Oestrogen helps the body to absorb calcium.

But diet alone will not preserve bone health. It is vital to do weight-bearing exercise that puts a stress on the bone, as this maintains bone density. Any type of activity in which we carry our own weight will help, such as walking, going upstairs, dancing and jogging, but we can increase the benefits with exercise designed specifically for this purpose. For more information about exercise or about courses run by agencies such as Extend (listed in chapter 10) see pages 38–53.

TOP TIPS FOR HEALTHY BONES

- Do weight-bearing exercises, such as running, jogging, walking uphill or climbing stairs. NB Activities such as swimming and cycling are not weight-bearing.
- Eat a balanced diet rich in calcium (found in milk and leafy green vegetables) and vitamin D.
- Cut out smoking completely and cut down on alcohol, tea and coffee, as caffeine inhibits your intake of calcium.
- Get a little sun. Sunlight makes our skin produce vitamin D, which in turn helps the body absorb calcium.
- Speak to your GP about your individual risk of osteoporosis and whether a scan is advisable to check this. Early treatment means better protection against a fracture in the future.

The people particularly at risk include those with a first-degree relative with osteoporosis; Caucasians and Asians; women who had an early menopause, and people on long-term steroids. Being a smoker or drinking more than the recommended levels of alcohol and taking no weight-bearing exercise are other important risk factors. It is also advisable to watch your weight – being under-weight increases the risk of osteoporosis and being slightly overweight might even be an advantage.

If you think you could be at risk, talk to your doctor, who may advise a DEXA scan, which measures bone density and can detect osteoporosis at an early stage (ordinary X-rays can do so only at a much later stage). Unfortunately, the availability of DEXA scans varies around the country; it may be easier to arrange one privately.

As far as treatment is concerned, in the past, many women at risk were advised to use hormone replacement therapy (HRT), as the

oestrogen it contains protects the bones, but this is no longer considered a first-line treatment for osteoporosis. You will need to discuss
with your doctor which of several alternative treatments is best suited
to helping you build up your bones. There is a school of thought, however, that suggests that since the risk of fracture is greatest at about
age 75, this may be the appropriate time of life to use HRT.

CANCER

Cancer is not one disease but a great many, a substantial number of
which can be cured. Although not all cancers are avoidable, some
are and there are definitely steps we can take to lower our risk.

Cancers are, in some ways, diseases of ageing, because they are
the result of cellular processes that go wrong, just as ageing itself is.
In the case of cancers, cells begin to divide abnormally and seem not
to know when to stop. The result is a malignant tumour which, if not
stopped in its tracks, has the potential to spread – through the bloodstream, for example – to other tissues. It is these secondary growths
that are most worrying because they are often harder to treat.

There are many risk factors for cancer, and diet is thought to be
linked to about one-third of them. As chapter 4 has shown, the antioxidants in fruit and vegetables offer us nature's best defence against
cancer and many other conditions. For example, onions and garlic
have been found to protect against a range of cancers, including cancers of the oesophagus, mouth, throat, colon, breast, ovary, prostate
and kidney. There is reasonable evidence that dietary fibre protects
against cancer of the colon and vegetables appear to be the best way
of getting the fibre for this purpose. Aspirin has been shown to protect against cancer of the colon and emerging evidence suggests that
it may also markedly reduce the risk of cancers of the skin, breast,
ovary and lung; the precise dosage varied somewhat across the different studies, but one aspirin a day or even less was frequently
sufficient.

In women, there is a link between obesity and cancers of the breast and womb, and there is also a link between obesity and cancer of the colon, so it is worth keeping the weight under control for these as well as many other reasons.

Smokers have a high risk of cancer – not only lung cancer but also cancer of the bladder, pancreas, stomach, oesophagus, throat and kidney. Some experts also believe that the benzene cigarettes contain is the cause of multiple myeloma, the primary cancer of the bones. Your risk of developing cancer begins to drop as soon as you stop smoking, so it is never too late. If you are finding it difficult to give up smoking, it is worth taking more exercise, which decreases the craving for nicotine, and massively increasing your intake of fruit and vegetables, as these will provide some protection.

Over-exposure to the sun can cause skin cancer, and because older people tan more slowly they have an increased risk. So, when tanking up on vitamin D from sunshine, go carefully – we should never expose ourselves to the sun long enough to burn.

It is important to remember that cancers can often be cured, at any age. If you discover a lump or something else that needs investigation, do not let fear delay your visit to the doctor. The earlier you start treatment, the more successful the outcome is likely to be – so much so that many healthcare professionals now view several types of cancer as a chronic disease.

OSTEOARTHRITIS

Osteoarthritis is so common as we get older that we may think it is the price we have to pay for our long lives. But it is not. There is much we can do to reduce our risk of this disabling condition.

Osteoarthritis, or inflammation of the joints, is most common in the knees, hips, hands, ankles, feet and spine. The cartilage at the ends of the bones becomes rough and thin, the connecting bone thickens and the surrounding tissues swell up. At its worst, osteoarthritis is

OSTEOARTHRITIS

This painful and potentially disabling condition, the most common joint disorder in the UK, is so common in later life that we tend to think of it as the inevitable result of wear and tear. But the causes are at least partly genetic, and there are exciting potential opportunities for 'fixing' arthritic joints without the need for radical surgery.

Normal joint   **Joint affected by osteoarthritis**

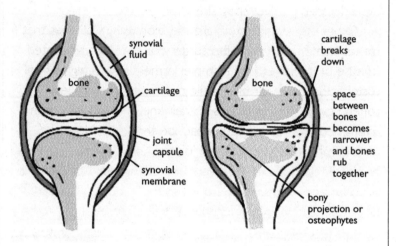

synovial fluid

bone

cartilage

joint capsule

synovial membrane

cartilage breaks down

bone

space between bones becomes narrower and bones rub together

bony projection or osteophytes

Areas affected

Osteoarthritis most commonly affects the knees, hips, feet, fingers and spine. The ends of the bones in these and other areas are protected by a layer of gristle called cartilage, which acts as a shock absorber when we put weight on the joint.

The smooth cartilage surface also allows the bone ends to move freely. In osteoarthritis patients, the cartilage does not function properly, the connecting bone thickens and the surrounding tissues swell up. At worst, the only treatment is radical surgery to replace the affected joint with an artificial one.

Osteoarthritis risk factors

The most obese people are six times more likely to develop osteoarthritis than those of ideal weight. One study estimated that the risk of knee osteoarthritis increases by 40 per cent for every 5kg of weight gained – fortunately, the risk also declines for every 5kg shed.

Other major risk factors are the 'biomechanical' ones that result from misaligned joints, surgery or trauma or repeated misuse of the joints. For example, farmers have a high risk of osteoarthritis in their hips, while professional footballers often develop osteoarthritis in their knees and hips, in both cases because of repeated impact on the joints. Normal exercise, however, benefits the joints.

There may also be some as yet unidentified hormonal risk factors: for example, loss of oestrogen after the menopause may increase the risk of osteoarthritis for women.

painful and disabling, though there is much sufferers can do to improve their quality of life.

The risk of developing osteoarthritis increases with age, particularly if you have a family history of it, or have injured a joint in the past. By the age of 65, 50 per cent of people have the disease in one or more of their joints, and about 10 per cent have some disability caused by it.

Other major risk factors are being overweight and taking insufficient exercise to keep the muscles strong. The more overweight we are, the higher our risk of getting osteoarthritis, especially in the knees. The most obese people are six times more at risk of this condition than those of ideal weight. If you already have osteoarthritis, the best way to help yourself is to reduce your weight – even shedding a few pounds will take some strain off damaged joints and prevent a worsening of the condition. And keeping active will help reduce pain and stiffness, hard though this may be to believe when you are the person in pain.

Muscle weakness also predisposes us to osteoarthritis. The idea that our joints 'wear out' with normal use is quite wrong – it is lack of use (or abuse) that puts joints at risk. This is yet another reason to take regular exercise, as chapter 3 explains. To avoid osteoarthritis we need both muscle-strengthening and aerobic exercise.

Suitable exercise also benefits people who already have osteoarthritis but this should be done under the supervision of a doctor or physiotherapist. However, it is recommended that we all exercise in footwear with thick, soft soles that act as a good shock absorber and that protects the joints.

Injury to the joints can happen as a result of repetitive impact. Professional footballers, for example, are at high risk of osteoarthritis in their knees. If you have had any type of joint injury – or surgery – it is all the more vital to exercise to keep the muscles strong.

About one and a half million people in the UK each year seek treatment for osteoarthritis from their GP, and an unknown number beyond that decide to self-medicate. Your doctor may suggest taking a painkiller such as paracetamol or a course of non-steroidal anti-inflammatory drugs such as ibuprofen, which are also available in cream or gel form.

The role of diet in preventing or controlling osteoarthritis is controversial. You may see all sorts of claims for certain food supplements but there is no good scientific evidence that any of these help. Nevertheless, a lot of people swear by glucosamine and chondroitin. Research on glucosamine is based on taking 1,500mg daily, but it is not advisable to take it if you have an allergy to seafood, as it is derived from shellfish.

Doctors recommend a well-balanced diet that contains plenty of fruit, vegetables and fish, particularly oily fish. Some people find that excluding certain foods from their diets is helpful but this is very individual and no general advice can be offered. ■

8

COMPLEMENTARY THERAPIES: THE SCIENTIFIC VERDICT

COMPLEMENTARY THERAPIES: THE SCIENTIFIC VERDICT

Science sometimes offers a new take on old discoveries. To what extent is this true for complementary medicine? As many as three in five of us use complementary therapy each year and sometimes it has been the GP who has provided the service or encouraged us to experiment. So what is the scientific evidence to support the claims made for these treatments?

TRIED AND TESTED REMEDIES OR EFFECTIVE PLACEBOS?

Many complementary therapies have been with us for millennia. The use of medicinal plants, for example, is probably as old as humankind itself, while acupuncture has been used and refined in China for at least 1,500 years. That these approaches have survived for so long says something about them, yet scientists have, on the whole, been slow to investigate their claims, or have dismissed any apparent successes as being the result of the 'placebo effect', whereby a dummy treatment produces positive results.

There is no doubt that the placebo effect plays an important role. Many practitioners say that the relationship between patient and therapist is a key factor in the healing process and good therapists are skilled at helping people to feel more positive about their health. However, these factors are important aspects of all medical treatment, as even orthodox practitioners recognise.

The result of this relative scientific neglect, however, is that there is little scientific evidence to support – or refute – the claims made for most complementary approaches. It is not even known whether some complementary therapies are safe, let alone effective. In 2001, the House of Lords Select Committee on Science and Technology conducted a review of complementary medicine and concluded that only osteopathy, chiropractic and acupuncture had good scientific evidence behind them. In the committee's view, the evidence for the effectiveness of herbal medicine and homeopathy was inconclusive or partial, while there was no scientific evidence at all to support any others.

Nevertheless, the government is anxious to ensure that the provision of complementary medicine is evidence-based and safe and is funding a range of projects through the Department of Health. One example involves the use of complementary and alternative medicine within palliative cancer care.

Other research is based on trying to design the sort of trial that will demonstrate evidence in a way comparable to the standard randomised controlled trial (RCT) used for conventional medicines. This can be tricky, particularly in the case of homeopathy, which in its pure form focuses on a single individual, whereas RCT results involve findings that emerge from studying large groups.

The lack of evidence is, of course, simply that. In a few years' time we will be able to report a different story. Many of the professional bodies are supporting research, while independent scientists and pharmaceutical companies are also conducting studies. In the USA a vast amount of research is in progress, some of it directly relevant to ageing. Most of this research focuses on clinical effectiveness but work is also being done on the basic physiology of the treatments.

At present we have only a vague understanding of what happens when, for example, an acupuncturist inserts the needles. But neuro-imaging suggests that certain acupuncture points do have distinct effects that cannot otherwise be obviously predicted. Functional magnetic resonance imaging (fMRI), which tracks the changes in blood flow that result from brain activity, is showing that acupuncture has a powerful and measurable effect on the brain. For example, it can reach the part which is involved in the perception of pain, suggesting that it may change the way we 'decide' whether something is painful or not. And points associated with hearing and vision – but quite distant from ears and eyes – do stimulate the visual and auditory cerebral areas respectively.

A recent book, *Complementary and Alternative Health: the scientific verdict on what really works* by Dr Steve Bratman in association with Professor Jayney Goddard, president of the UK's Complementary Medical Association, covers the study findings to date that validate – or not, as the case may be – the use of complementary approaches in specific circumstances; it looks at what we know and do not know about popular complementary treatments, states their strengths and weaknesses, and compares them with conventional treatments for the same condition.

Also, a major study at the University of Westminster (as yet unpublished) has been looking at the interactions between conventional and complementary medications. This is intended to help doctors when advising us on whether it is safe to mix the two.

THE MAIN THERAPIES, AND CURRENT SCIENTIFIC ASSESSMENTS

Acupuncture uses fine needles, which are inserted in the skin to stimulate special points on the body and is used to treat a wide range of conditions. We know that acupuncture increases the body's release of natural painkillers – endorphin and serotonin – and that acupuncture can affect homeostasis, the body's mechanism for keeping our metabolism in equilibrium. So far the effect on different systems, such as the immune system, is only poorly understood. However, there is good evidence that acupuncture is effective in the treatment of postoperative nausea (as is acupressure) and some evidence that it may help lower back pain, some other types of pain and migraine. Major studies of the effects on back pain and migraine are now in progress in the UK, as is a study of acupuncture in the rehabilitation of stroke patients, where early findings are encouraging.

Aromatherapy is based on the alleged healing power of plant oils, which may be massaged into the skin, inhaled or used in the bath. Anecdotally it is said to induce a feeling of well-being. Aromatherapy massage uses massage techniques to relieve tension and improve circulation and there is some evidence that this is effective in reducing anxiety in short-term settings such as intensive care. A placebo-controlled trial of melissa (lemon balm) aromatherapy showed a 35 per cent reduction in agitation and increased social interaction in dementia patients.

Herbal medicine has always attracted some scientific interest and many well-known drugs are plant-derived: for example, digoxin from foxgloves and morphine from poppies. Only a minority of plants have been studied, however, and many traditional remedies have still to be investigated.

We also need to know much more about the interactions of herbal remedies and prescribed drugs as there are worrying indications that some do not mix.

The following are some of the herbs that scientists believe to be effective and safe, or which appear to merit further study.

- St John's wort (*Hypericum perforatum*) is a safe and effective treatment (if taken as the only treatment) for mild to moderate depression. It may also help fatigue, possibly because fatigue is a common aspect of depression.
- *Ginkgo biloba* may be effective in relieving the symptoms of dementia and it may also support memory in all older people. More work is needed to confirm this.
- To date, studies on ginger as a remedy for nausea and vomiting have shown contradictory results.
- Phytodolor (a standardised extract of *Populus tremula* and other herbs) is as effective as low-dose synthetic drugs in relieving rheumatic pain.

- Horse chestnut seed extract can alleviate the symptoms of varicose veins.
- Tea tree oil may be effective against fungal infections such as athlete's foot and deserves further study.
- Vegetables from the allium family (onions and garlic) may protect against certain cancers if eaten regularly, especially cancers of the digestive tract, though further studies need to be done. However, it is no longer thought that garlic reduces cholesterol levels, as was previously claimed.

Homeopathy is based on the principle that 'like can be cured with like'. Illness is treated with low-dose preparations that induce similar symptoms: for example, hay fever may be treated with a remedy based on onions. The House of Lords Committee was not convinced about the scientific evidence but others say there is some evidence that homeopathy is effective against illnesses with an allergic component, such as asthma, hay fever and rhinitis, and it may also combat influenza. Further research is needed into whether it is effective in osteoarthritis as there is some promising evidence.

Osteopathy, a relatively new therapy, uses manipulation of the bones and other parts of the musculoskeletal system to restore and maintain mechanical function.

Chiropractic is used to treat similar conditions. Based on the evidence, both this treatment and osteopathy are now recommended by the Royal College of General Practitioners for the treatment of lower back pain. There is also some evidence that they can help some types of headache.

Reflexology is the massage and compression of reflex areas in the feet, or sometimes hands, and it is used to treat a variety of conditions. There is no good scientific evidence that it is effective. However, in Denmark, where reflexology is very popular and is offered by many employers, research has shown that it can reduce levels of illness in the workplace.

TEMPTED TO TRY?

If you would like to try one of these therapies it is vital to go to a trained and reputable practitioner. Some therapies are completely unregulated: for example, anyone can call themselves an acupuncturist or an aromatherapist. You can contact the Complementary Medical Association or the appropriate professional body (www.web-health.co.uk/professional bodies provides a helpful list) to check your nearest qualified practitioners, or you may be able to get advice from your GP. You may even find that your GP has a qualification in, say, homeopathy or offers some complementary therapies through the surgery.

You also need to be aware that no treatment is risk-free. We have already mentioned possible interactions between herbal remedies and prescribed drugs. There have been some cases of stroke and other injuries as a result of chiropractic and some adverse reactions to acupuncture, though these are very rare.

Whatever therapy you try, it is important to see it as a complement to whatever your GP is offering and not a substitute for it. There is no scientific evidence that any complementary therapies are effective at diagnosing health problems and it can be dangerous to rely wholly on them as treatments. Always discuss them with your GP. ■

9

SCIENTISTS' TOP TIPS FOR AGEING WELL

SCIENTISTS' TOP TIPS FOR AGEING WELL

1 TAKE MORE EXERCISE

Studies have shown that 'exercise deficiency syndrome' is the biggest risk we face as we get older. Exercise is key to a healthy cardiovascular system. It helps us keep our arteries elastic and lowers our blood pressure. It also helps mood and prevents depression. It is worth remembering that even moderate levels of physical activity are valuable. Try to walk for 20 minutes a day. For maximum health it is best to vary the type of exercise. Weight-bearing exercise – such as walking or going upstairs – is important, as it puts stress on bones, helping to maintain bone density. However, to prevent falls you need to follow exercises that improve your dynamic balance, such as ballroom dancing, yoga or *t'ai chi*.

2 STOP SMOKING NOW!

Not only is smoking associated with a number of health risks, including cancer, heart disease, stroke and respiratory problems, but it also slows down your rate of healing, decreases your muscle tone and adversely affects bone health. Remember, it is never too late to quit and start experiencing the benefits. Call the NHS smoking helpline (see chapter 10) for help and advice.

3 KEEP SOCIALLY AND MENTALLY ACTIVE

Having a strong network of family and friends, and lots of purposeful activity is vital to health as we get older. It is widely recognised that older people who have regular mental stimulation, whether from good conversation or setting themselves mental challenges, appear to maintain their cognitive abilities better. Play cards, do crosswords, invite friends and family round or do whatever else it takes to keep your brain active.

4 DRINK MORE WATER

Many older people are slightly dehydrated, which not only leads to constipation, but can also cause mental confusion and urinary tract infections. Try to drink water rather than fizzy drinks, which contain lots of sugar or artificial sweeteners, and avoid too much tea and coffee. The problem with caffeinated drinks is that they are diuretics, so they will increase the amount of water you excrete and make you more dehydrated.

5 GET OUTDOORS AS OFTEN AS POSSIBLE

About 10–20 minutes of sunshine a day helps you produce vitamin D, which is needed for bone health. But moderation is important. While sunshine helps your bones and boosts your sense of well-being, over-exposure destroys skin elasticity, causes age spots and can lead to skin cancer. For this reason it is important to wear a sun block, and follow the simple rule of never exposing yourself to the sun for long enough to burn.

6 MAKE SURE YOU HAVE GOOD NUTRITION AND EAT A BALANCED DIET THAT INCLUDES PLENTY OF FRUIT AND VEGETABLES

These are nature's anti-ageing remedy, protecting us from many of the diseases associated with later life. Our calorie requirements become slightly lower as we age, because we are less active, making it important to eat foods that have lots of essential nutrients in proportion to their calories, such as whole grains, fresh vegetables and fruits and legumes. Eat fewer 'treat' foods with empty calories, such as cakes, biscuits, sweets and crisps.

7 IF YOU DRINK ALCOHOL, DRINK LITTLE AND OFTEN

Studies have shown that people who regularly drink small amounts of alcohol tend to live longer than people who do not drink at all. This is because modest amounts of alcohol protect against cardiovascular disease.

Alcohol can also help to prevent gallstones, prostate problems and cognitive impairment. But moderation is important: maximum benefit is achieved by drinking one or two units of alcohol a day – for men; women should drink less. Drinking any more may result in health problems. Alcohol can weaken your immune system, affect your cognitive abilities and increase your risk of falling. It can also increase the risk of cardiovascular diseases, some cancers and liver and pancreatic disease.

8 MAKE YOUR HOME SAFE

Check your house and garden for possible dangers, including trailing cables, loose mats and uneven paving slabs that could trip you up and result in falls and broken bones. Increase the level of lighting everywhere – especially on the stairs – so that you can see properly.

9 SEE YOUR GP, DENTIST AND OPTICIAN REGULARLY

Do not put up with health problems on the grounds of age or assume that nothing can be done. Get your blood pressure checked annually and, if it is found to be high and requires medication, make sure that you check it regularly: out-of-control blood pressure can result in serious medical conditions such as stroke. Knowing your cholesterol level and keeping it low is also a good thing.

10 TRY TO BE POSITIVE

Studies show that having a positive outlook on life actually boosts our immune system. Also, be positive about your wants and needs too – studies show that longevity appears to be linked to a determination to stay in control. It appears that people who find life comprehensible and manageable have better health outcomes than those who do not. ■

10
SOURCES OF FURTHER INFORMATION

HELP THE AGED

207–221 Pentonville Road
London
N1 9UZ
Tel: 020 7278 1114
Fax: 020 7239 1489
Email: info@helptheaged.org.uk
Website: www.helptheaged.org.uk
International charity working to improve the lives of older people. Funded by individuals, companies and trusts, it carries out research, campaigns for improvements in policy and practice and provides practical services to help older people stay independent.

The Charity includes:

SeniorLine
Freephone 0808 800 6565 (Northern Ireland 0808 808 7575), providing free, confidential and impartial advice on benefits, care and housing issues

SeniorLink
Tel: 0845 053 2306, a home telephone-response service that connects users with a response centre for emergency assistance or reassurance (24 hours)

and the biomedical research programme
Research into Ageing
(see page 189).

OTHER ORGANISATIONS AND WEBSITES

Alzheimer Scotland
22 Drumsheugh Gardens
Edinburgh
EH3 7RN
Tel: 0131 243 1453
Helpline: 0808 808 3000
Website: www.alzscot.org

Alzheimer's Society

Devon House
58 St Katharine's Way
London
E1W 1JX
Helpline: 0845 300 0336 (8.30am–6.30pm Mon–Fri)
Website: www.alzheimers.org.uk
Alzheimer's Society and Alzheimer Scotland offer specialist advice for people with dementia, their carers and families.

The Andropause Society

20/20 Harley Street
London
W1G 9PH
Tel: 020 7636 8283
Website: www.andropause.org.uk
The Society for the Study of Androgen Deficiency (androgen = testosterone) offers information and help in the use of testosterone for the treatment of the 'male menopause'.

Arthritis Care

18 Stephenson Way
London
NW1 2HD
Tel: 0845 600 6868
Helpline: 0808 800 4050 (10am–4pm)
Website: www.arthritiscare.org.uk

Arthritis Research Campaign

Copeman House
St Mary's Court
St Mary's Gate
Chesterfield
Derbyshire
S41 7TD
Tel: 0870 850 5000
Website: www.arc.org.uk

British Heart Foundation

14 Fitzhardinge Street
London

W1H 6DH
Heart information line: 08450 70 80 70
(8am–6pm Mon–Fri)
Website: www.bhf.org.uk

British Nutrition Foundation
High Holborn House
52–54 High Holborn
London
WC1V 6RQ
Tel: 020 7404 6504
Fax: 020 7404 6747
Email: postbox@nutrition.org.uk
Website: www.nutrition.org.uk

BTCV
Sedum House
Mallard Way
Potteric Carr
Doncaster
DN4 8DB
Tel: 01302 388 888
Fax: 01302 311 531
Email: information@btcv.org.uk
Website: www.btcv.org.uk
The BTCV Green Gym® scheme aims to inspire people to improve their
health and the environment at the same time. It offers the opportunity to
'work out' in the open air through local, practical environmental or gardening
work. Contact BTCV to find the Green Gym centre nearest to you.

Cancerbackup
3 Bath Place
Rivington Street
London
EC2A 3JR
Tel. (freephone helpline): 0808 800 1234
Website: www.cancerbackup.org.uk
High-quality, up-to-date information, practical advice and support for cancer
patients and their families.

Chest, Heart and Stroke Scotland
65 North Castle Street
Edinburgh
EH2 3LT
Advice line: 0845 077 6000
Website: www.chss.org.uk
Specialist advice and guidance for people who have had a stroke, their carers
and families. (See also Stroke Association.)

Complementary Medical Association
CMA Chief Administrator
Blackcleuch
Teviothead
Hawick
TD9 0PU
Tel: 0845 129 8434
Email: admin@the-CMA.org.uk
Website: www.the-cma.org.uk
Refers medical professionals and members of the public to qualified, insured
practitioners who adhere to the organisation's strict code of ethics and
disciplinary procedure.
See also Webhealth.

The Continence Foundation
307 Hatton Square
16 Baldwins Gardens
London
EC1N 7RJ
Tel: 020 7404 6875
Helpline 0845 345 0165
Website: www.continence-foundation.org.uk
Advice and information on continence problems. See also InContact.

Department of Health
Tel: 0800 155 5455
For details of health benefits and healthcare claim forms, or help with the
cost of getting to hospital.

Diabetes UK
Macleod House
10 Parkway

London
NW1 7AA
Tel: 020 7424 1000
Careline: 0845 120 2960
Website: www.diabetes.org.uk

Digital Unite
Website: www.digitalunite.net
Offers computer training and is especially keen to include hard-to-reach people, such as care home residents.

Do It
First floor
50 Featherstone Street
London
EC1Y 8RT
Tel: 020 7250 5700
Fax: 020 7250 3695
Website: www.do-it.org.uk
Volunteering opportunities. Part of Youthnet, a registered charity.

Emotion
Head Office
48 Earlsway
Teesside Industrial Estate
Thornaby-on-Tees
Tees Valley
TS17 9JU
Tel: 01642 807090
Fax: 01642 652299
Email: sales@emotionshoes.co.uk
Website: www.emotionshoes.co.uk
Fashionable shoes and boots for wider feet and calves.

Extend
2 Place Farm
Wheathampstead
Hertfordshire
AL4 8SB
Tel/fax: 01582 832760
Email: admin@extend.org.uk

Website: www.extend.org.uk
Provides recreational movement to music for men and women aged over 60 and for less able people of all ages. Aims to promote health, increase mobility and independence, improve strength, co-ordination and balance and to counteract loneliness and isolation, thereby enhancing quality of life.

Hearing Concern
95 Gray's Inn Road
London
WC1X 8TX
Helpline (telephone and textphone): 0845 0744 600
Website: www.hearingconcern.org.uk

Home Heat Helpline
Tel: 0800 33 66 99 (9am–8pm Mon–Fri, 9am–3pm Sat)
Minicom: 0800 027 2122
This freephone service offers practical energy advice from trained advisers to people concerned about paying their energy bills, or to those calling on behalf of a friend or relative.

InContact
Satra Innovation Park
Rockingham Road
Kettering
Northants
NN16 9JH
Tel: 0870 770 3246
Website: www.incontact.org
Advice and information on continence problems.
See also Continence Foundation.

Keep Fit Association
1 Grove House
Foundry Lane
Horsham
West Sussex
RH13 5PL
Tel: 01403 266000
Fax: 01403 266111
Email: kfa@keepfit.org.uk
Website: www.keepfit.org.uk

Macmillan CancerLine

Tel: 0808 808 2020 (9am–10pm Mon–Fri)
Email: cancerline@macmillan.org.uk
For information on cancer care and Macmillan nurses.

Malehealth

c/o The Men's Health Forum
Tavistock House
Tavistock Square
London
WC1H 9HR
Website: www.malehealth.co.uk
Free, impartial information from the website run by the
Men's Health Forum and partially funded by the NHS.

The Marigold Clinic

The Royal London Homeopathic Hospital
60 Great Ormond Street
London
WC1N 3HR
Tel: 020 7391 8873
Bunion treatment referrals.

Menopause Amarant Trust

Tel. (helpline): 01293 413000 (11am–6pm Mon–Fri)
Website: www.amarantmenopausetrust.org.uk

Mind, the Mental Health Charity

15–19 Broadway
London
E15 4BQ
Info line: 0845 766 0163
Website: www.mind.org.uk

National Osteoporosis Society

Camerton
Bath
BA2 0PJ
Tel: 0845 130 3076
Helpline: 0845 450 0230
Website: www.nos.org.uk

NHS Choices

Website: www.nhs.uk
New online service with sections on living well, an A–Z of conditions and treatments and a search facility for NHS services.

NHS Direct/NHS24

Tel: 0845 46 47 (calls charged at local rates)
Websites: www.nhsdirect.nhs.uk; www.nhsdirect.wales.nhs.uk; www.nhs24.com (Scotland)
A 24-hour nurse-led helpline providing confidential healthcare advice on information on health concerns, local health services, self-help and support organisations. Calls cost a maximum of 5p a minute from BT landlines, but call costs from mobiles and other networks may vary.

NHS Smoking Helpline

Tel: 0800 169 0169 (10am–11pm every day)
Website: www.gosmokefree.co.uk
If you are feeling under pressure or under scrutiny and wish to talk to someone about giving up smoking without risk of being judged, this helpline's trained advisers will listen and offer help.

Open University

Website: www.open.ac.uk/openlearn
An interactive learning site offering courses for both professional purposes and leisure free of charge.

Parkinson's Disease Society

215 Vauxhall Bridge Road
London
SW1V 1EJ
Helpline: 0808 800 0303
Website: www.parkinsons.org.uk
Specialist advice and guidance for people with Parkinson's, their carers and families.

Partially Sighted Society

7–9 Bennetthorpe
Doncaster
DN2 6AA
Tel: 0844 477 4966 (9.30am–4.30pm Mon–Fri)
Fax: 0844 477 4969
Website: (via) www.patient.co.uk

The Prostate Cancer Charity
First floor
Cambridge House
100 Cambridge Grove
Hammersmith
London
W6 0LE
Tel: 020 8222 7622
Helpline: 0800 074 8383
Fax: 020 8222 7639
Email: info@prostate-cancer.org.uk
Website: www.prostate-cancer.org.uk

RNIB (Royal National Institute of Blind People)
105 Judd Street
London
WC1H 9NE
Tel: 020 7388 1266
Helpline: 0845 766 9999
Website: www.rnib.org.uk

RNID
19–23 Featherstone Street
London
EC1Y 8SL
Helpline: 0808 808 0123
5-minute hearing check: 0845 600 5555
Textphone: 0808 808 9000
Tinnitus helpline: 0808 808 6666
Website: www.rnid.org.uk
Formerly the Royal National Institute for Deaf People.

Silver Surfers
Website: www.silversurfers.net
For anyone of over 50 who wants to find out about the internet and
how to use it.

Society of Chiropodists and Podiatrists
Head Office
1 Fellmonger's Path
Tower Bridge Road
London
SE1 3LY
Tel: 020 7234 8620
Fax: 0845 450 3721
Website: www.feetforlife.org

Stroke Association
Stroke House
240 City Road
London EC1V 2PR
Tel: 0845 3033 100
Website: www.stroke.org.uk
(For Scotland, see Chest, Heart and Stroke Scotland.)

University of the Third Age (U3A)
National Office
19 East Street
Bornley
Kent
BR1 1QE
Tel: 020 8466 6139
Website: www.u3a-info.co.uk

Webhealth
354 Mansfield Road
Nottingham
NG5 2EF
Tel: 0115 960 8855
Website: www.webhealth.co.uk
Information on 'natural health' (complementary therapies) and a
'practitioners search' facility that will help you to locate your nearest
qualified practitioners.

YMCA
Website: www.ymca.org.uk
For finding exercise classes with seniors-qualified instructors.

FURTHER READING
Dr Dawn's Health Check: everything your doctor doesn't have time to tell you by
 Dr Dawn Harper (Mitchell Beazley, 2007).
The Testosterone Revolution by Dr Malcolm Carruthers, MD (Thorsons, 2001).

Exercise books and videos for older people
Strength and Balance Exercises for Healthy Ageing
In a convenient wire-bound, flip-over format, this collection of strength and
balance exercises can safely be undertaken by older people at home. It was
produced by Help the Aged in collaboration with Wandsworth Primary
Care Trust and Camden Active Health Team (London Borough of Camden).
(Help the Aged, 2006)

Be Strong, Be Steady (video)
A programme of chair-based and standing exercises devised specifically for
older people with mobility difficulties. Done regularly, these exercises will
strengthen muscles, increase flexibility and improve balance, all of which will
help to reduce the risk of falls. (Help the Aged, 2004, 2005)
English plus Cantonese/Punjabi/Bengali editions. Running time 58 minutes

Step to the Future (video, DVD)
Aerobic endurance and strength exercises including standing, chair-based and
floor routines, all devised specially for older people and set to a music track.
(Help the Aged, 2006) (DVD contains options for English subtitles and Hindi
voiceover) Running time 90 minutes

Menopause
The New Natural Alternatives to HRT by Marilyn Glenville, PhD (Kyle Cathie,
 2003). Provides a detailed account of what is happening to the body during
 the menopause, and sensible advice on handling the change.
The Menopause Diet by Theresa Cheung in conjunction with Professor Adam
 Balen, Professor of Reproductive Medicine at Leeds General Hospital
 (Vermilion, 2007).

Both books take as their starting point that adjusting eating habits may be
enough to restore balance to wayward hormones.

Complementary therapies
Complementary and Alternative Health: the scientific verdict on what really works
 by Dr Steve Bratman in association with Professor Jayney Goddard (Collins
 in association with Complementary Medical Association, 2007).
Complementary Medicine for Dummies by Jacqueline Young (John Wiley, 2007).

INDEX

ACKNOWLEDGEMENTS

Dr Elizabeth Breeze of the ELSA Study (English Longitudinal Study of Ageing), University College London

Dr Malcolm Carruthers, President, The Andropause Society, London

Professor Jayney Goddard, President, The Complementary Medical Association, London

Dr Dawn Skelton, Reader in Ageing and Health in the School of Health and Social Care, Glasgow Caledonian University

Professor Tim Skerry, School of Medicine and Biological Sciences, University of Sheffield

How to Thrive Past 55 was originally researched and written by Hilary Todd and published by Research into Ageing. Many research scientists and clinicians generously contributed their time and expertise to the publication: Professor Sir John Grimley Evans, Department of Clinical Geratology, University of Oxford; Professor Tom Kirkwood, Professor Oliver James, Professor Rose Anne Kenny, Professor John O'Brien, Dr Julia Newton, Dr Jo Harbison, Professor Elaine Perry, Professor Gary Ford, Institute for Ageing and Health, University of Newcastle; Dr Dawn Skelton, Senior Research Fellow at the UCL Institute of Human Performance, Royal National Orthopaedic Hospital, Stanmore; Dr Susan Jebb and Dr Beckie Lang, MRC Human Nutrition Research, University of Cambridge; Dr Derek Browne, former GP and founder of the Age Concern Ageing Well campaign; Dr Neil Pendleton, Clinical Gerontology, University of Manchester; Professor Simon Lovestone, Institute of Psychiatry; Professor Carol Brayne, Institute of Public Health, University of Cambridge; Professor E. Ernst, Department of Complementary Medicine, University of Exeter; Dr Mark Bovey, Complementary Health Studies Programme, Department of Education, University of Exeter; Dr Anne McArdle, Muscle Research Centre, Department of Medicine, University of Liverpool; Dr Pippa Tyrrell, Director of Stroke Services, Hope Hospital, Manchester; Dr David Gunnell, Department of Social Medicine, University of Bristol; Dr Michael Hastings, Department of Anatomy, University of Cambridge; Professor Michael Doherty, University of Nottingham.

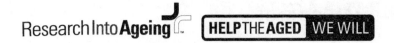

Research Into **Ageing** **HELP THE AGED** WE WILL

RESEARCH INTO AGEING

Research into Ageing was founded in 1976. It is now a special trust within Help the Aged and a member of the Association of Medical Research Charities. The Charity raises funds to support the best and most-needed biomedical research that will improve understanding of health in later life and lead to better treatments and ways of preventing health problems.

Understanding what is happening to the body as we get older and why it is more likely to break down or wear out is the first step to improving health and independence. This is why we support research into the biology of ageing as well as into the specific diseases that become more common as we get older.

We fund research into the most common illnesses affecting older people, including mobility problems, Alzheimer's disease, osteoporosis and stroke. This makes us different from most other medical research charities because we do not concentrate on one disease or one part of the body, but take a broad approach and fund research that will help to improve the quality of later life. Biomedical research is one of the most powerful tools available for making a difference to the quality of later life.

To make a donation, or for particular information about individual giving, please contact Customer Relations on 020 7239 1982 or write to us at Research into Ageing, Help the Aged, 207–221 Pentonville Road, London N1 9UZ.

HELP THE AGED

Help the Aged is an international charity dedicated to creating a world where older people can live their lives free from poverty, isolation, neglect and ageism. We also work to prevent deprivation among future generations of older people, by improving prospects for employment, health and well-being so that dependence in later life is reduced.

The Charity's unique understanding of older people's needs enables it to raise public awareness of issues affecting older people in the UK and overseas, campaign for changes in policy and practice nationally and regionally, and provide practical support to help disadvantaged older people live independent lives. Independent of government, it is funded by individuals, companies and trusts. It also operates advice lines, publishes information and guidance, and runs a nationwide network of charity shops.

With your support, we can achieve even more. Could **you** help **us** to help older people, by:
- donating unwanted goods to your local Help the Aged shop?
- recycling your old mobile phone, toner cartridges or glasses to raise vital funds?
- selling raffle tickets or contributing to one of our appeals?
- making a regular donation by direct debit or online at www.helptheaged.org.uk?
- applying for a Help the Aged credit card?
- signing up to Sponsor a Grandparent overseas?

To find out more about supporting Help the Aged, visit **www.helptheaged.org.uk**